CW01663840

Smart aids to live well

Staying healthy with assistive technology

Dr Ruth Chambers

Lee Owen

Alex Rowley

Paul Edden

Nachi Chockalingam

Copyright

Cartoons by John Byrne. http://johnbyrnecartoons.com

Date of publication - September 2021

Disclaimer

Whilst every effort has been made to include accurate and up-to-date information about legal requirements, IT infrastructure and other resources such as hyperlinked websites - knowledge and understanding are constantly evolving and being updated. The assistive technology items that are included in the various chapters in this handbook are just examples and are not recommendations of the different forms of digital aids that are readily available. Therefore, please use the content of this book to learn more about how you can adopt or enhance your use of digital healthcare and assistive tech aids for your own health and wellbeing and weigh up the choices, information and guidance for your own circumstances. The content is not a substitute for clinical advice from the doctors and nurses and carers who look after you, or for national advice and guidance from professional or regulatory organisations. Inclusion of named agencies, websites, companies, services or publications in this book does not constitute a recommendation or endorsement.

Contents

Authors

The five co-authors bring in the experience and wisdom of a long practising doctor, academics, care providers and technology experts.

Professor Ruth Chambers OBE

Ruth has been a family doctor for 40+ years. She is an Honorary Professor at Staffordshire University and also Keele University. Ruth's previous research interests have focused on self care, effective ways of working, stress in health professionals, and many other health related themes in various healthcare settings – most recently technology enabled care services in the NHS. She is also co-director of Alegre Ltd, the company signposting 'My Health Kit' aids. Ruth has worked with the Royal College of General Practitioners, Department of Health/NHS England and other healthcare organisations on various projects over the last three decades. Most of Ruth's work has related to improving the quality of delivery of healthcare. Ruth has written 73 books, mainly for health professionals, but three have been for the general public on stress, heart disease and back pain; four books have been translated into other languages – Japanese, Italian and Korean.

Lee Owen

Lee is Community Development Coordinator with Staffordshire County Council. He has over 16 years experience working within the Staffordshire Health and Social care sector. Initially working in customer care services, he has spent the last 10 years as a community development coordinator, working with community groups, health and social care teams, exploring various ways of maintaining independent living. Lee has actively promoted the use of assistive and digital technologies which are readily available on the high street and online, that can help to support people and their carers. Pre-COVID, Lee regularly attended community events to promote independent living, but during the pandemic has linked to people virtually. Currently Lee is working on developing a web-based tool that can help to find assistive and digital technology solutions for people who are struggling with daily living tasks.

Alex Rowley

Alex is Director and Chief Technical Officer of Wavemaker CIC. With a professional background spanning 20 years, Alex has a significant amount of experience with technology. His skills encompass technical aspects of networking infrastructure, equipment deployment and management, training, support, advice and guidance. Furthermore, Alex's digital and graphic design skills, twinned with a high attention to detail, help to bridge these two areas when working with a client. Alex has an in-depth knowledge of the challenges that relate to the education and training sector. He is passionate about helping to steer change, as an individual and representative of Wavemaker. The organisation's core aim is to empower individuals with the knowledge, skills and confidence needed to utilise technology in order to enhance and improve their lives.

Paul Edden

Paul is Managing Director of Home Instead, based in Northern Staffordshire. With a professional background in telephony and technology totalling nearly 40 years, Paul is skilled in all areas of telephony equipment, project management, training and sales. Paul also gained much international experience as a business consultant for the Concert organisation, a joint venture between BT and MCI. Taking a right angle turn in his career, Paul was invited to assist the master franchisor for Home Instead to establish this US model of care provision into the UK in 2005. After 5 years at the master franchise organisation, which had grown under his guidance from one to 44 offices in the UK, Paul and his wife Sandra decided to open their own franchised office serving Newcastle-under-Lyme and Stoke-on-Trent. Currently, this office now employs over 70 local people and provides care for over 100 people across the area. Paul is passionate about providing compassionate, quality, relationship-led care for his clients and has of late become engaged in various projects surrounding the installation of subtle intelligent sensors within clients' homes to further ensure their safety whilst they are alone. Paul believes that technology cannot replace physical care, and nor should it. But he does believe that some products can enhance the overall care experience, ensuring that Mum or Dad can continue to live in their own home, whilst loved ones are reassured of their wellbeing and safety.

Professor Nachiappan Chockalingam

Nachi Chockalingam is a Fellow of the Institute of Physics and Engineering in Medicine. He is the Director of the Centre for Biomechanics and Rehabilitation Technologies at Staffordshire University and also an Affiliate Professor at the Faculty of Health Sciences, University of Malta, a Visiting Professor at the Department of Sports Medicine and Arthroscopy, Sri Ramachandra University in Chennai and a Guest Professor at Guangzhou Sport University, China. He has received research funding from various international bodies including the European Commission and British Council and has over 650 research outputs, including over 200 full research manuscripts. He led a project in collaboration with the World Health Organisation and the International Society for Prosthetics and Orthotics to support the development of Standards for Prosthetics and Orthotics Service Provision. He is involved in charitable and non-profit organisations to help the wider global community on healthy ageing and assistive technology to aid mobility. He is also co-director of Alegre Ltd, the company signposting 'My Health Kit' aids.

Preface

We have written this handbook to provide 'ordinary' people with a wide range of advice & ideas about using various tech aids to help them (or a loved one) stay healthy - that they can apply to their own circumstances. So read this book & realise how you can use smart aids in your own everyday life – so then you'll live healthily, be as mobile as possible, stay safe & independent at home – and yes, you can do this!

Technology is your friend when it comes to managing your health and wellbeing. There is a wealth of knowledge, information and experience available at our fingertips which has revolutionised the way we live our lives. Our tips are frequently scattered in each chapter to help to give you ideas of ways to use assistive technology and digital services for yourself or your loved ones. Not everything will work for everyone - it's about being aware of the options and choosing what is right for you or your family. Each chapter contains useful information relating to the use of simple, relatively low cost assistive technology to promote a person's health, independence and wellbeing. These items are either free (like many of the trusted apps featured in every chapter) or affordable and readily available in the retail market and so can be purchased by the individual themselves or by their family/carer etc. Please be mindful that we are not endorsing any particular product but simply making people aware of what is available, how they can access it, how it can be used and might benefit them, or their loved one.

People who can benefit from assistive technology are anyone and everyone, but particularly:

- those with chronic disease or long-term conditions by supporting their self-care (see Chapter 2).
- those who will benefit from lifestyle support for healthy living through activity monitoring (see Chapters 3, 4, 5, 6).
- older people living alone – it helps to minimise the risks in their own homes, increasing their confidence relating to trips and security (see Chapter 7).
- people with physical disabilities by providing remote control devices with risk management to provide easier access to emergency services in the event of an accident like a fall (see Chapter 7).

- people with increased frailty by providing a safety net of support and long-term monitoring of the progression of their health condition and wellbeing (see Chapter 7).
- people with back or other muscle or joint problems, to help them to combat pain and build or maintain their strength (see Chapters 8 and 9).
- people with sensory impairments such as loss of vision or hearing by associated sensors to help compensate for their reduced senses and minimise risks in their everyday living e.g. with a range of automatic home-based sensors (see Chapter 10).
- people with early or moderate dementia – it helps with reminders and sensors to detect any dangerous situations they are in at home, and maximises their independence through electronic aids and emergency detection (see Chapter 11).
- people with mental health problems such as anxiety, depression or stress by providing support at times of crisis if they are connected to a remote community service and help them to comply with taking their medication regularly and doing other therapies (see Chapter 13).

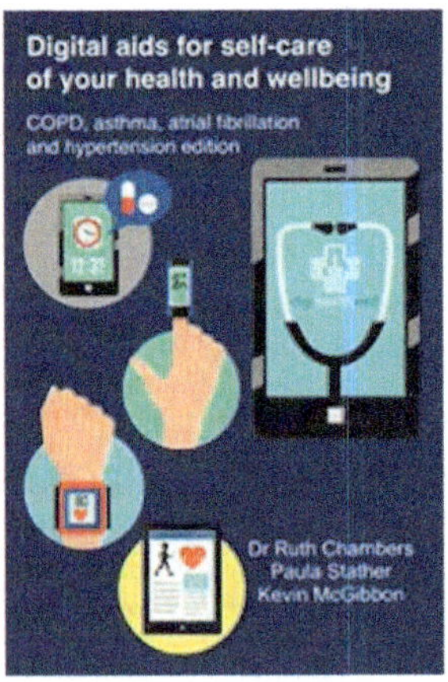

Take a look at our parallel handbook: Chambers R, Stather P, McGibbon K: Digital aids for self-care of your health and wellbeing. The book relays digital tips and suggestions for health conditions like asthma, raised blood pressure, the irregular heart rhythm atrial fibrillation, and chronic obstructive pulmonary disease (COPD).
You can purchase an Amazon kindle or paperback copy at

https://www.amazon.co.uk/Digital-aids-self-care-health-wellbeing/dp/1838397787

Chapter 1. How technology can assist your wellbeing and independence

Top tips:

1. Technology can assist people with health and wellbeing problems to self-manage their conditions better and engage with clinicians, or friends and family.
2. Find out how easy and useful digital aids can be, matched to the purpose you want it for.
3. Technology can never replace physical care by person-to-person interaction - and nor should it.

Technology is increasingly integrated into most people's everyday lives. Many people use technology for entertainment, food preparation, banking, communication, travel and transport. The effects of the COVID pandemic have been to push many more people to use digital technology like their smartphone or tablet in different ways, such as for booking appointments at their GP's surgery or video consultation instead of a face to face meeting with a doctor or nurse.

Four out of five adults in the UK now own a smartphone – that's around 95% of people aged 16-24 years old, though fewer older people use one – probably only about half of those aged 55 years or older. A smartphone gives people computing power with access to a simple touch screen, a high quality camera and microphone, cellular voice and text messaging and high speed connections to the internet (often their main way of getting online).

The people most likely to feel digitally excluded from being able to interact with healthcare professionals or make appointments or send requests to general practice or hospital staff are older people, those with disabilities or who have limited English language skills. Sometimes it is about not having the skills, but also not having the technology (can't afford the equipment and/or Wi-Fi access to the internet, or their technology such as mobile phones are too old, or don't want it) to go online or make video calls. Ofcom reports that around 6% of homes in the UK (that's about 1.5million) have no internet access.

The COVID pandemic made this even more difficult as people were expected to shift to remote and digital health care from their usual face to face care or interactions, and people reluctant or unable to use modern technology feel left out and isolated. A recent report from the Ida Lovelace Institute found that a fifth of people in the UK do not have access to a smartphone and as many as 14% do not have broadband internet.

In the UK the average life expectancy of someone at the age of 65 years old, is around 18 more years for men and 21 more years for women - although this does vary greatly between those from affluent and deprived backgrounds. A healthy person aged 65 years old can expect to be without a long-standing illness or disability for around 10 years.
With increasing age they may start slowing down, have less energy and take longer to undertake daily activities – so this is when they need to recognise and take action to gain more control of their lives.
And technology can assist them with that.

So enhancing self-management of your long-term health and wellbeing means that you must:

- gain a realistic understanding of any health condition(s) that you have (including doing your own research on the internet) and understand what actions you can take to slow down the progression of your disease(s) and prevent worsening of the symptoms.
- learn how to look after yourself - especially your feet, eyes, mental wellbeing and socialising, keeping active, having a healthy lifestyle such as avoiding excessive alcohol or quitting smoking and a good diet.
- know what helpful resources are available such as assistive technology or self-care support networks for example.
- remember to take your prescribed medication and adhere to other recommended treatments and actions.

Many doctors and nurses do offer their patients the chance to use technology as part of their usual service of care – including interactive text messaging, apps if they've got health conditions, video-consultation with a doctor or nurse, and updates via social media such as Facebook or

WhatsApp Groups. Remote interactions with a doctor or nurse are much easier for people if that means that they don't need to travel from work or home to their general practice or hospital, or find a car parking space – so long as they have the tech equipment with them or at home, to join in. Over recent times there has been a rapid shift to remote consultations between a patient and their doctor or nurse - though this is still most likely to be by text messaging and telephone contacts rather than by other remote connections such as video-consultation and email. But for those patients who are not digitally savvy, many of whom are older people who are more likely to have multiple health conditions, this has created more health inequalities from their lack of ready access to primary care and their lack of digital skills in the use of apps or video-consultation.

Technology has revolutionised the way that we live now and is reshaping our lives. It is becoming normal to use digital technology to promote people's health and social wellbeing, matching their needs with digital solutions – for prevention of their deterioration (e.g. tech reminders to take medication regularly), aiding their treatment (e.g. wearable technology measuring blood sugar or someone's heart rate) and supporting their safety and independence (e.g. with light sensors or personal digital assistant).

Digital solutions can empower people to self-manage their health and wellbeing and connect them with their families and carers in intelligent ways – to enhance their wellbeing. But this does not replace personal contact and care from clinicians like doctors and nurses. The more that people are confident in using technology and can access the right equipment with a stable internet connection, the more sustainable the national health and care system will be in future.

Some older people are comfortable with using an electronic tablet but not as comfortable in using their smartphone in the same way.
For example, they might use the internet on their tablet regularly but would never access it through their phone because of their fears around inputting their personal information on the internet – and others having access to their personal details.

Wearable technology

In a never-ending world of constant developments, the range and use of wearable technology for self-monitoring of your health is moving fast. People who purchase wearable tech are usually health conscious and want to understand their body better and take more control of their health. Wearable devices integrate sensors that gather data about a person's activity or other aspects of their health, into a device that they carry in their pocket, or wear on their wrist or waist.

Some products display data for that person on their device; others send the information elsewhere as a form of telecare, for an overall analysis by a centre set up to do so. So a smart watch might relay whether a wearer has fallen down, or is experiencing involuntary movements as in Parkinson's disease; and if set up to do so, contact the specialist service in that event.

The personal fitness app market has flourished over the past years. They usually capture past trends in related biometric measures as well as current performance, and enable their owner to set targets, so that data can motivate them to sustain positive behaviour like increased daily exercise activity. Smart watches tend to have additional functionality too, with extra features such as calendars, messages and email notifications. Most require pairing with a smartphone to be fully functional, which makes them more expensive. The Apple Watch can detect whether a person's irregular pulse rate is likely to be due to the medical condition, atrial fibrillation (though it would still need to be confirmed by their doctor or nurse).

You need to be aware of some of the risks with wearable technology too as well as the benefits. Some people are not able to understand or operate their kit, some tech devices (e.g. those without a CE mark) may generate data that is unreliable, or some self-monitoring devices may induce competitive urges which are not healthy – such as losing too much weight or undue lowering of their heart rate. So you should be aware of the limitations of every piece of technology and not become over-reliant on it.

Assistive technology

There is a wide array of technology available today that can help people to feel safer in their home. Smart devices can allow you to monitor and control your home setting from the palm of your hand using a smartphone or tablet, or by your voice when using a smart speaker. Popular items in the home include smart light bulbs, plug sockets, doorbells and security cameras. Smart speakers can help someone to feel less isolated and keep them connected with friends and family too.

Assistive technology includes any device or system that allows a person to perform a task that they would otherwise be unable to do, or increases the ease and safety with which they can perform the task. So this might include substantial equipment like stair lifts, clever technology like exit sensors that can detect if a vulnerable person leaves their home, or small aids like non-slip mats. There is no one magic product that will suit everybody in all situations. Using assistive technology is appropriate for everyone and should not be considered as simply a direct replacement for personal contact and family/carers' support. It enables people to lead their own lives, keep mobile and stay independent. Assistive technology is not just for the elderly or infirm – an increasing number of households have a voice activated assistant or smart security aids like a video doorbell.

As people go through life, they may need some extra help to stay independent and safe in their own homes. Buying some simple daily living equipment or technology can really help them to manage everyday tasks on their own. Assistive technology includes any item, piece of equipment, product or system, whether acquired commercially, off the shelf, modified or customised, that is used to increase, maintain or improve the functional capabilities of individuals with cognitive, physical and/or communication disabilities. Assistive products or devices range from low to high tech versions for personal medical treatment, training in skills, personal care and protection, personal mobility, housekeeping, communication and information, handling objects and devices, as well as splints and artificial limbs, and furnishings and adaptations to homes and othersettings.

Assistive technology maintains or improves people's well-being and independence too. This might include jar openers, bath seats or stair lifts, and electronic sensors and aids that make their home environment safer with home adaptations as well as newer technologies. A lot of these items are more affordable than people think and can be purchased cheaply from a local high street shop, supermarkets and on the internet, or from specialist equipment shops. Self-monitoring of blood pressure may give a truer estimate of a person's usual blood pressure than readings by a doctor in the surgery and remote exchange of a person's valid blood pressure readings, enabling a clinician to make an intelligent analysis; associated advice or modify their treatment, may save time for health professionals and patients.

Using community alarms and other telecare technology can help people of any age and ability to live independently, safely and securely in their own home. The assistive tech devices can be linked to a triage system where alerts can be relayed directly to social or health care teams, or family or friends. Such telecare services might be based on a combination of alarms, sensors (like motion sensors and door locks) with monitoring activities designed to raise a call for help if the pattern of someone's behaviour who lives there, changes. It can give family and friends peace of mind that they can be contacted in an emergency.
A community alarm or care call system can link the person at home to a 24-hour monitoring centre through a landline telephone link which can be activated by the service user pressing a button worn as a wristband or pendant etc.
This then triggers an alarm call via a base unit to the monitoring centre. The centre will know their details and the trained and skilled operators can offer support or help to organise the care they need. Any sensors or alerting devices are wirelessly connected and communicate with the centre via radio signals; this can be used around the home and within a short distance away in the gardens of the home. Read more about this in the section on *Sensors* below.

Smart plugs have a wide range of uses. They can:

- keep your home secure – for instance when you're away from home, you can use a smart plug to turn a lamp on at your home so it looks as if you're there.
- start cooking your evening meal whilst you're at work by switching your slow cooker on via your smart plug an hour or two before you expect to arrive home.

- enable carers to oversee a loved one without being in the same home by remotely checking what appliance operated by a smart plug is switched on, using their own smart phone app.
- set up *Alexa* by linking the plug to an Echo Show or Echo Dot to turn it on when asked to do so.

Sensors

Sensors can identify remotely when and where a carer's input is required (e.g. if their loved one has a fall detected), rather than carers or family members visiting someone 'just in case'.

The future of sensors also includes passive data gathering, with meaningful interpretation including:

- necklaces that can monitor heart function and check the amount of fluid in your lungs, and headbands that can capture brain waves.
- wireless and wearable sensors that can track vital signs without touch.
- medications that will be digitised to ensure that they have been taken as prescribed.
- socks and shoes to analyse gait and alert a carer as to whether an elderly family member is unsteady and at risk of falling.
- for people with diabetes, Google's smart contact lens gives a real-time measurement of blood glucose levels, by assessing glucose levels in a person's tears and transmitting this data to a smartphone or other external device. With the added benefit of abolishing painful finger pricks it will become a much more convenient method for patients to use to control their diabetes.

MySense sensors

This system uses a series of sensors around a person's house to detect when they get up, where they go around the house, how often they flush the toilet or fill the kettle up or open the fridge etc. These sensor reports are relayed to a machine learning system that builds up a pattern of the person's daily living activities. If the machine recognises an aberration in the person's daily living habits it flags this up to pre-agreed professionals or carers who can intervene in case those pattern changes indicate initial signs in deterioration of the person's condition.

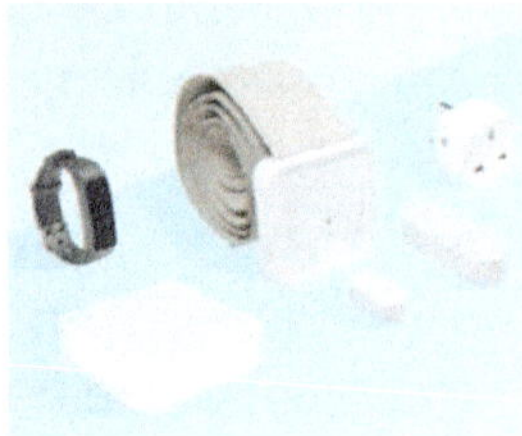

So this sensor system can replace face to face interaction from a family member or social carer where it's not needed, or makes the home environment safer where it is needed.

Advances in technology have made it possible to monitor a person's movement and action within their own home on a constant basis. If the sensors fitted within the home are paired with intelligent software, it is possible to gain insights into the person's normal daily routine over time. The intelligent software can gather the triggers from the various sensors fitted around the home and use the information received to build a *trend* of the person's normal activity. Hence it is also possible to report *unusual* activity or behaviour and raise prompts or alarms, as necessary.

Whilst technology can't replace the human touch and benefits of person-to-person care, it can enhance an older person's life. In particular, technology can provide comfort and reassurance for remote family members that older loved ones are safe and doing well at home.
With the use of a few small but subtle sensors, it is possible to stay connected to your loved ones, know if something is not quite right and continue to care, even when you're not physically there.

The *system* learns what normal looks like for any one individual person and then looks for any changes which might show that things are not as they should be.

Any changes can be shared over the internet with care providers and with family members who are looking out for Mum or Dad's wellbeing via an app on their mobile phones and/or an email or text message.

The format of devices will vary depending on an individual's needs, but a typical example of an installation could be:

- **Smart plugs** that are installed on standard devices across the home, from lamps to TVs, kettles to fridges, and everything in between. These plugs can spot if Mum or Dad is eating and drinking regularly, staying active throughout the day and still watches the news at 6pm each evening - so there is no need to worry.
- **Temperature sensors** to check that Mum or Dad is comfortable at home in the correct setting, so that they can avoid problems caused by cold weather.
- **Activity tracking sensors** to provide reassurance that Mum or Dad went to bed at their usual time and stayed there until their normal rising time. They might monitor their number of visits to the bathroom during the night - which could provide an early indication of problems such as urine infections etc.

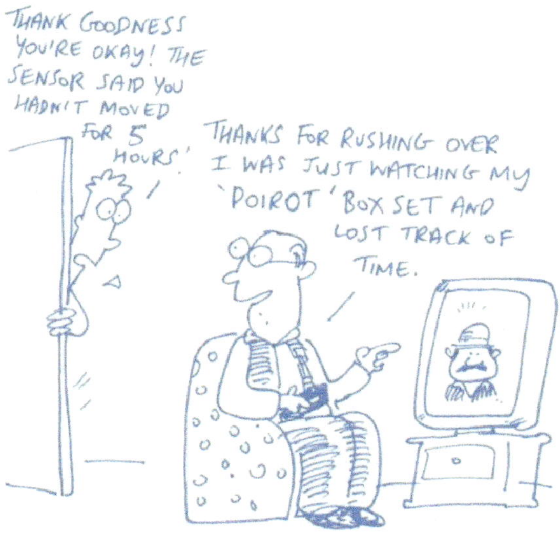
THANK GOODNESS YOU'RE OKAY! THE SENSOR SAID YOU HADN'T MOVED FOR 5 HOURS!
THANKS FOR RUSHING OVER I WAS JUST WATCHING MY 'POIROT' BOX SET AND LOST TRACK OF TIME.

These systems are designed and formatted to send an alert to a family member or carer if there is a suspected problem in the home – for risk areas such as falls, inactivity, malnutrition and lack of sufficient fluid intake. By remotely monitoring an older person's activity and other factors in their home, the technology helps to keep them safe and independent. It also provides reassurance to family and friends who may not be able to call round in person as often as they would like. Combined with intelligent software, these devices can help to prevent a problem happening before it occurs.

The following list of available sensors and their possible uses can be customised to fit well with your, or your loved one's, needs:

- Hydration and nutrition: fridge door sensors keep track of meal times; smart plugs identify if the kettle or microwave is turned on/off.
- Bed or chair sensors: positioned under a mattress or the seat of a chair, can detect if someone moves or falls from their bed or chair, or fails to get out of bed, for example.
- Movement sensors: detect when a person is moving around their home or if they are immobile for too long.
- Fall detectors: send an alert if they sense a sudden jolt or downward movement by the person being monitored.
- Door sensors: let you know when someone leaves or enters the home. An alert could be sent if this happens at an unexpected time of the day, or if the front door is left open for an extended period.
- GPS tracking devices: keep track of someone when they are out and about. They can be attached to clothing or even built into a pair of shoes.
- Flood detectors: sensors in the kitchen or bathroom can spot if water is overflowing or a tap has been left on. They can send an alert or even turn off the water supply directly.
- Heat/temperature sensors: by detecting extreme temperatures in the home, they can spot a fire hazard or avoid the risk of a person suffering hypothermia.

- Incontinence sensor: provides a warning if a person urinates or vomits whilst in bed.
- Medication dispensers and reminders: help to remind someone to take their medication, dispense the correct pills and keep track of what is taken and when.
- Smoke or gas detectors: like standard household alarms these emit a loud alarm if triggered but can also be set up to transmit an alert to a monitoring centre or a family member.
- Wearable alarm pendants: pressing a button sends an alert to a monitoring centre or carer.

Many of these products can enhance someone's overall care experience, ensuring that they can continue to live in their own home, whilst loved ones are reassured of their wellbeing. Information gathered by the sensors and analysed by intelligent software allows interventions when needed, identifies early signs of older age illnesses, and can trigger help to ensure that the person is eating, drinking and exercising properly.

Then that person should be:

- Safe: activity sensors show if a regular routine is being followed, flagging when something unexpected occurs.
- Well: sensors around the home and in the kitchen can demonstrate that they are staying nourished and hydrated throughout the day, particularly crucial for the elderly.
- Connected: we cannot always be there for our loved ones, but it doesn't mean having to be disconnected. Relatives and carers can have peace of mind knowing that intelligent monitoring will notify them when something is out of place. Wherever families are based, they can be connected and reassured.

If you are struggling to find solutions to a daily living task that you are struggling with, there are internet sites that offer impartial advice on forms of assistive technologies, for example **AskSARA**.

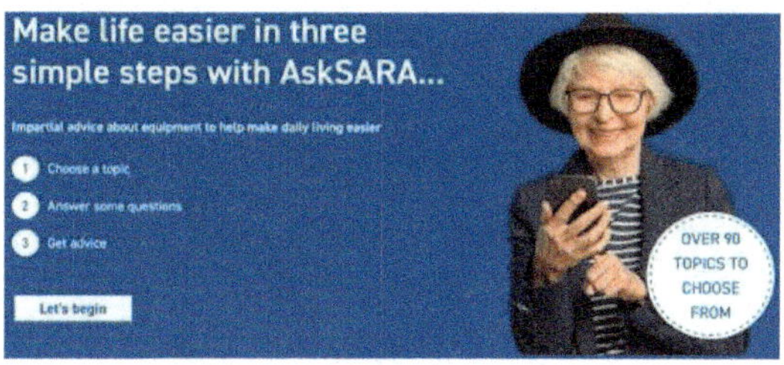
Make life easier in three
simple steps with AskSARA...
Impartial advice about equipment to help make daily living easier
1 Choose a topic
2 Answer some questions
3 Get advice
Let's begin
OVER 90 TOPICS TO CHOOSE FROM

This online self-help guide provides expert advice and information on products and equipment for older and disabled people that is easy to use at home: https://carersuk.livingmadeeasy.org.uk/about-ask-sara

You can access Staffordshire County Council's ***Happy at Home*** website which involves an interactive home. Your journey starts with you picking a room where you're struggling with a daily living task, and then transporting you to a series of ideas and solutions that could possibly help you to overcome your difficulties and challenges. The innovative *Happy at Home* house highlights the range of simple and affordable assistive technology equipment available, such as help to prepare food, get washed or dressed or feel safer around your home. There is a library of video demonstrations of assistive technology products that lets you compare a wide choice of solutions. People can explore the online interactive house and find out more at: www.staffordshire.gov.uk/happyathome

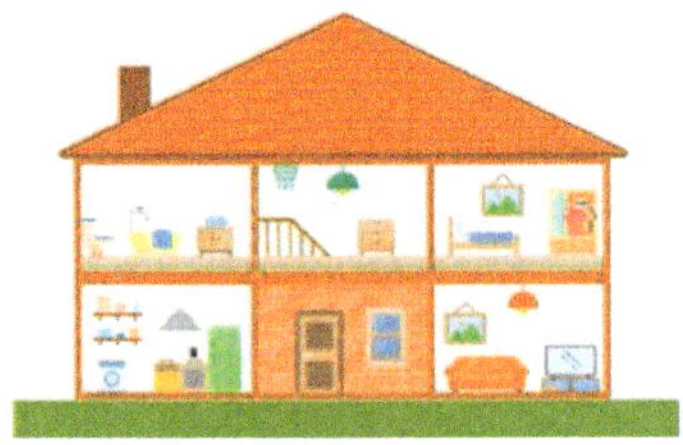

Have a look too at Telford and Wrekin Council's virtual house link below – it offers virtual tours of various rooms in the home; if you click on a piece of tech (highlighted by circles) it tells you what it is, what it does, how much it costs and where to buy it, linking through to their independent living centre:

https://www.telford.gov.uk/info/20792/independent_living_centre_ilc_and_virtual_house/5264/virtual_house_tour

Smartphones

The smartphone is more than just a phone - it's a powerful portable computer. These devices not only allow you to make calls, access the internet and view video streaming services, but are also capable of having dedicated computer programmes (or apps) installed on them that can offer a tailored experience suited to a particular need. A key feature of an app is its ability to send notifications to your phone - a great way to keep engaged with the app content and continue to use it to reach your goals, say.

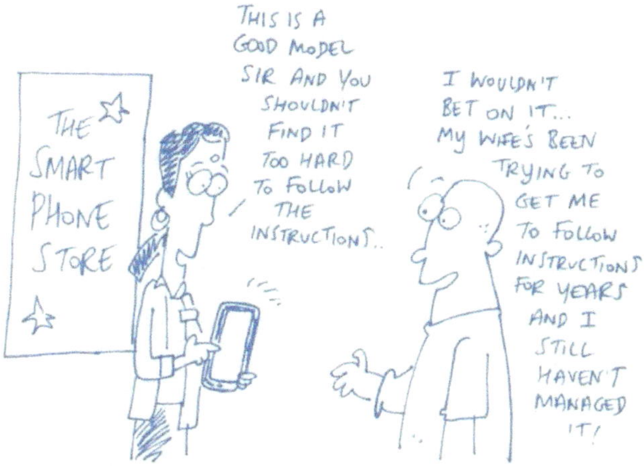
THIS IS A GOOD MODEL SIR AND YOU SHOULDN'T FIND IT TOO HARD TO FOLLOW THE INSTRUCTIONS..
I WOULDN'T BET ON IT... MY WIFE'S BEEN TRYING TO GET ME TO FOLLOW INSTRUCTIONS FOR YEARS AND I STILL HAVEN'T MANAGED IT!
THE SMART PHONE STORE

Smartphones are cited as the most important device for accessing the internet at home or elsewhere among all adults, rather than a computer (laptop or desktop) - with online text messaging being much more popular for daily use by online adults than emailing is.

A smartphone has a touch screen, high-quality camera, short and long range wireless connections, cellular voice and text messaging service with high speed connections to the internet. Many younger people use their smartphone as their exclusive means to get online, rather than using a tablet, iPad, computer or kindle. Google's operating system for smartphones and tablets are called *Android.* So Android phones and tablets are an alternative to an Apple iPhone and iPad.

Smartphones vary, but for most, you'll need to do fairly similar things to get them to work. 'Swiping' – moving your finger quickly across the screen upwards or to the right will probably change what your screen looks like, and bring a few symbols (icons) to view.

Icons may vary slightly.

You have probably learnt to **make calls** using your smartphone.

You can store people's numbers in '**contacts'** Tap the icon to open the list, and then the + sign to add a new person's details. A keyboard will appear when you need it.

Tap **message** icons like these to open up your text messages, and to write a message. You may need to 'compose' one or tap the icon. If you have a friend's name in your 'contacts' list, you can usually type the name into the 'recipient' box, and the message will find the right person's details. To write a message, tap the message box – it may be quite small but will open up as you type. A keyboard appears, and you can tap letters to create the words you want to write. Sometimes the phone will suggest words which you can click on, to speed up your writing.

The arrow symbol at the bottom left of the keyboard changes writing to **capital letters**, and another key lets you write **numbers or symbols**,

Use the thick arrow with the cross key to **delete** a previous letter, and the kinked arrow to **end a paragraph or 'enter'**

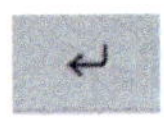

To **send** your text message, press 'send' or an icon which looks similar to this:

To find out more about using a computer (your phone is a small but powerful computer), go to the *learnmyway* website. To do this, go to your internet browser on your screen (you may need to swipe up or to the right) and tap it. A page should open up with a box into which you can write www.learnmyway.com You'll need to register to join the free course, so tap the word 'register', and then complete your details.

The course will help you to use a computer, and your phone is very similar, but without a separate keyboard.

There are also apps already in your phone, or more available from the App Store (if you have an iPhone) or Google Play Store.

Apps

An app (short for 'application') is a type of programme used on all smartphones, tablets and newer versions of Windows. They are installed on your device through an app store, like Apple's App Store, the Google Play Store, and Windows 10 Microsoft Store.

Health apps can enhance your understanding of your health condition and empower you to manage your health or be more aware of your lifestyle habits (good and bad!) and the associated effects. They can provide information, help you to record readings (e.g. your blood pressure), encourage activities or other good behaviour, and even arrange feedback for you from health professionals.

There are loads of apps out there – hundreds for each health condition. When downloading apps, always check the description, user rating (usually out of 5 stars) and reviews to ascertain whether the app is good and will be of use for you. You're best to choose one that's been recommended by your doctor or nurse or someone you trust if it relates to your health. Otherwise the app might guide you to do the wrong thing with managing your health. Some are free, some are costly.

The NHS Apps library has accredited, recommended apps for a variety of health conditions available at: https://www.nhs.uk/apps-library/

Other health apps can be found directly through the Apple App Store and Android Play Store. Health charities like the British Lung Foundation and British Heart Foundation also provide useful trusted apps. App stores feature thousands of health and wellbeing apps. If your phone's too basic for loading up the apps that you want, maybe a family member will load it on to theirs and let you use it (though take care if you do not want to share confidential details).

With the use of a smartphone or tablet device you can download apps to assist you with self-care and management of your health at home. Downloading an app after you have read some of other people's reviews e.g. on the NHS Apps Store, will give you an idea as to whether it is relevant to your needs. But be aware that some apps can incur a cost – if so, you'll need to decide if that cost is worthwhile for what you need the app for, and if it is affordable.

Personal digital assistants

Relatively new in recent years, but becoming increasingly popular, are smart speakers or personal digital assistants. They come in a range of shapes and sizes, some with screens, some without. Ones with a screen offer greater functionality and accessibility, and are favoured by the majority of users. Smart speakers are available from a range of manufacturers but the leading ones are Google's Nest and Amazon's Alexa. Smart speakers are a great way to find out information quickly and easily, using only your voice. Breaking down the barriers to using technology, they offer a rich experience and can do many things from offering news and information, to reminding you to take your medication.

Personal digital assistant devices can be used to:

- set reminders for taking your medication, or other daily tasks
- provide information e.g. exercise routines and facts about health conditions
- improve your access to the internet by using voice control to make calls
- answer your questions (search the internet and find you the answer)
- tell you the time
- alert you with alarms
- tell you the weather forecast
- check your calendar
- tell you what's in the news
- play music that you request.

Some features on a digital assistant will require additional service subscriptions which vary in cost. These are generally monthly payments and cannot be purchased as a 'one-off'. The Amazon Alexa is a smart speaker that retrieves and plays information and multimedia. Depending on the model, this is either played through the speaker or through a display screen and a speaker. Alexa is controlled using your voice with no physical interaction necessary. You do not even need to be beside the device, as it can receive commands from across the room (say 10 yards away). This is unlike smartphones, tablets and computers, which require the use of a touch screen, keyboard or mouse.

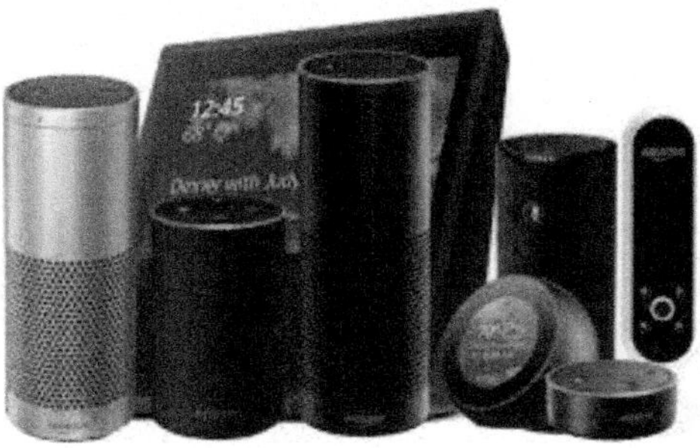

Example of Amazon smart speakers available

Online resources

It's estimated that over 1.7 billion websites exist across the world, so that's a fair bit of information available. Websites range from simply providing basic information, to in-depth, interactive and engaging content.

QR codes

At the end of most chapters in this handbook you will find QR codes which link to a website, a video and/or an app. A QR (Quick Response) code is rather like a barcode, but instead of being made up of lines it consists of lots of small squares in a seemingly random pattern.
QR codes can be scanned quickly and easily by using your smartphone's camera, which will then display the corresponding link, which once tapped will open the webpage, video or app.

QR codes will save you having to type in a website address manually.

For example, one way of finding the 'Active 10 Walking tracker' app on a phone or tablet is to copy laboriously the following into the bar at the top of a search page:

For an Apple phone or iPad : https://apps.apple.com/gb/app/one-you-active-10-walking-tracker/id1204295312

For an Android or Google device:
https://play.google.com/store/apps/details?id=uk.ac.shef.oak.pheactiveten

To save you having to do this, the 'QR code' which your smartphone or tablet can read can take you automatically to where you can see it:

Apple AppStore:

Google Play Store:

They are easy to use, on most modern smartphones.
Simply open the camera and point it at the QR code and the phone will automatically recognise the QR code.

A message will pop up asking if you'd like to visit the link contained within it, and then transfer you to the appropriate site.

If you have an older smartphone and this doesn't work you will need to download an app from the app store. Search for 'free QR code reader' app and install it as you would any other app. Don't be put off by this – it will be worth it in the end! Here are the instructions:

1 Look for the Google Play Store symbol on your smartphone. It will look something like this:
2 Tap it, and it will produce a screen with several app pictures, and at the top a box saying 'search for apps & games'. Tap this box, and a keyboard will appear on the screen.

3 Type 'qr code reader' and you will see a selection – choose any one that looks OK – they will have ratings beside them, (max 5.0 so 4.7 or 4.8 is good); some will advertise that they are free, and there will be a number of times other people will have downloaded it. The fact that four million people have done this, gives you confidence that you are not alone in choosing it.
4 Tap the one you want, and it will appear on the screen, with an option to 'install'. Click on the green bar, and once it has been downloaded to your phone or tablet, you can 'open' it.
5 Usually you will see a frame which you need to line up over the QR code, and after that, either everything happens automatically – the website opens, or you find you are at the app you wanted – magic! Or you may just need to tap a box which says 'WEB' – then the magic happens!

Then open the newly installed app and this will allow you to use QR codes.

But do note that downloading apps will use up some of your data allowance which is usually included in your mobile phone package, so it is better to download apps using Wi-Fi if you are downloading complicated apps. If you don't know how to connect your phone to your Wi-Fi, you could ask for help, or try following these instructions:

- Make sure your Wi-Fi is turned on, and you know what it is called (e.g. BT 5472 / Sky 72CO5 / TALKTALK 78G7F9). Note also the password you need to use.
- Go to the settings on your phone / tablet (it probably looks like this):

- Tap it, and then look for 'Connections', then 'Wi-Fi'.
- Tap the switch on the screen so that it is active.

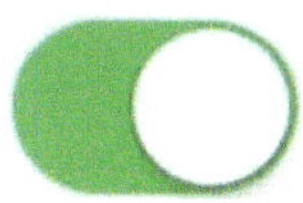

- Choose your Wi-Fi, if there is more than one, and when asked, enter your password, then click 'connect' or 'auto connect'.

Video streaming: services such as **YouTube** and **Vimeo** have been around for many years, but in more recent years have become even easier to access due to their integration with smart TVs and set-top-boxes. They offer videos covering many topics. The chances are that someone has already created a video offering tips, support and guidance. Many good content creators operate their own channel, and post videos at regular intervals. Subscribing to their channel allows you to see the latest content available, and makes it easier to browse at a later date.

Digital skills to underpin the technology reshaping our lives

The term 'digital' is confusing. Many people don't realise that the technology they use in their everyday lives can be applied to helping them to understand their health condition(s) and staying well.

Ann thought that digital health referred to the health of her laptop and had brought this along to be fixed when she attended a local self-help group at her local library; whereas the library leader meant group members should use their smartphone, tablet or laptop in different ways for their own personal wellbeing!

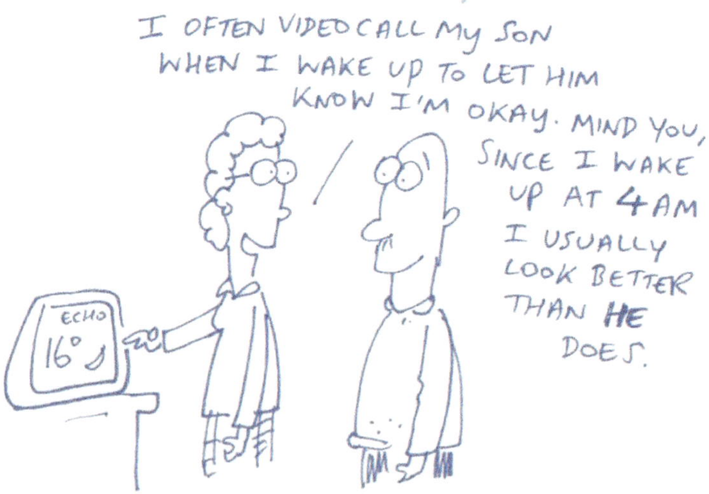
I OFTEN VIDEO CALL MY SON WHEN I WAKE UP TO LET HIM KNOW I'M OKAY. MIND YOU, SINCE I WAKE UP AT 4AM I USUALLY LOOK BETTER THAN HE DOES.
ECHO
16°

Using social media and the internet carries risks of which people need to be aware, so that they understand how to identify and mitigate these to keep their health and personal data safe. They need to realise that their personal data may be collected by commercial providers through their wearables and apps that they use. And thus they should pick trusted apps to upload to their phone or tablet. The essential digital skills that someone needs these days to promote their health and wellbeing are:

1. Communicating: able to go online, and engage in video-consultation or online groups like WhatsApp, text messaging.
2. Accessing health services: able to access their own medical records via the app that their general practice uses, and complete online consultation forms to e.g. order a repeat prescription or make a GP appointment.
3. Problem solving: using trusted websites and apps to compare their own symptoms and signs with recommended advice and guidance for next steps, including prevention and self-care such as improving their lifestyle habits.
4. Being safe online: keep personal accounts secure with safe passwords; and being aware of potential scams.

Password tips

Many people struggle with choosing a password. You want a password that you will remember but that a hacker won't be able to figure out. Don't use the same password for all of your accounts, and take especial care of your email account. If your email account is compromised then a hacker could use that to gain access to your other accounts, by requesting a password reset. Think of your email account as a master key to all of your other online accounts.

In an ideal world you would use a unique password for every account you have, but in everyday practice that is hard to manage and remember. Therefore, you're best to categorise your accounts into groups (see below), using the same password for all the accounts in the group, but a different password for each group. That way, if one of the sites you use has a data leak and your password is exposed, you only need to change the passwords on the individual accounts that are in the same group.

Example groupings of accounts:

Group	Description
Group 1	Email account
Group 2	Well known (trusted) e-commerce sites such as eBay, Amazon
Group 3	Social media accounts
Group 4	Media streaming services such as Spotify and Netflix
Group 5	Any other accounts

Avoid obvious passwords; some of the easiest passwords to remember are also some of the least secure. Try to avoid using passwords that are also:

- your partner's name
- your child's name
- your pet's name
- your home address.

While these types of passwords are easy to remember, the information is also fairly simple for a hacker to find out.

In some cases, such as your address information, it may even be in public record. If a hacker manages to get into your social media account, they can probably also learn the names of those close to you. Passwords that others commonly use are also bad choices. They are among the first that a hacker would try to gain access to your account with. Some of the worst passwords that people use (and that should be avoided) are:

- 123456
- abc123
- password

- welcome
- dates of birth
- other family members' names
- current partner's name
- place of birth.

The best passwords are random and contain various types of characters.

For example, a password that contains upper and lowercase letters, numbers and symbols is harder to hack than a password consisting of all letters or numbers. The longer the password, the harder it is to hack. Passwords should be at least eight characters long. Some experts recommend using as many as twelve characters even. Avoid stand-alone online password generators since the site may be trying to harvest passwords.

Some of the characteristics that make your password hard to guess, also make it harder to remember. That's why it's important to come up with a secure way to store your passwords.

Whenever possible, avoid:

- using your email password on a public computer. If you do use your password on a public device, clear the cache and memory afterwards. You may also wish to change your password.

- keeping your password on your person. Writing your passwords on a slip of paper and keeping it in your wallet can be a problem if your wallet is lost or stolen.

- storing your password in an unprotected document.
  It's common for users to create Word or Excel password lists. This is not a secure practice. The trouble is anyone who accesses your machine can open these documents.

To create a strong password:

- use three words or more (or more than 8 characters)
- include a symbol
- use upper and lower case letters
- include numbers.

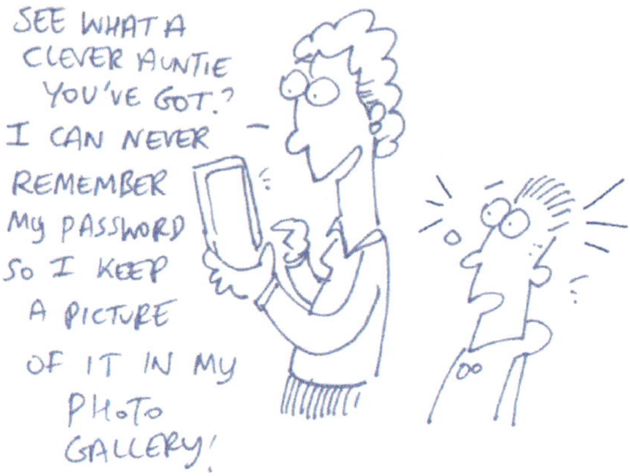
SEE WHAT A CLEVER AUNTIE YOU'VE GOT? I CAN NEVER REMEMBER MY PASSWORD SO I KEEP A PICTURE OF IT IN MY PHOTO GALLERY!

Case studies

Alan – how a personal digital assistant has brightened his life
Using his Alexa Echo Show as a personal digital assistant has helped Alan to feel safer in his home; for instance with reminders set to lock doors, smart sockets and light bulbs that can be controlled by his voice, and when his doorbell rings he can check who's at the door without getting up. That's all very useful as Alan is disabled after a stroke and uses a walking frame to move about the house.
Until recently he'd felt really lonely being stuck at home as it is difficult for him to get out and about and this adversely impacted on his mental wellbeing. Through his personal digital assistant he has connected with friends again and does video calls with his daughter or son everyday as they both live more than 50 miles away...so now Alan would describe himself as being more optimistic and happy about how the next stage of his life will go.

Hilda – how smart home monitoring has helped

Hilda (a 90 year-old) has four children who each live at least an hour away. Hilda received three care visits a week.
Hilda's family and her carer were concerned that she was not active enough, although she was fiercely independent and insisted that she could cope at home alone. Smart home monitoring was identified as the solution that would establish if any further help was needed. Sadly, the monitoring system confirmed that Hilda had lost much of her ability to be independent.
The technology showed that she was using her microwave less, stayed in bed longer, and rarely left the house. The family saw these changes in the activity graph available through the app they used. After discussion with Hilda and her family, care visits were increased, giving her more help at mealtimes. She even rekindled her love of cooking. Now, family members have visibility of Hilda's daily activities when she is alone and give her additional support if it is needed. Alison, Hilda's daughter says: "Previously, it was difficult knowing my Mum's lifestyle from dawn until dusk, and that made it hard to know how much care she required.
We can now match the support she needs with the right level of care. My family and I have so much peace of mind with the information provided by this technology. It means we can be extra sure that she is in safe hands."

Questions & Answers

Q1. I've heard of the term 'smart plug' and a friend told me he's bought one to switch his slow cooker on a few hours before he leaves work so his meal's ready when he arrives home. What else can a smart plug do – I'm thinking of buying one (or even a few!)?

A. You could use a smart plug to turn a lamp on when you're away on holiday so it looks as if you're still staying at home – many people find that useful to help keep their home safe. You could use a smart plug to turn your electric blanket on a short while before you go to bed, to save you clambering upstairs to do it – easy peasy!

A smart plug can be linked with an Alexa voice controlled option so that the user can turn that light or electric blanket on without having to reach over to the plug. You can buy a batch of smart plugs which you can set up round an elderly relative's house, set up to help you monitor what they are doing to ensure that they are safe and pursuing their usual daily activities.

Q2. I like the idea of using a mobile health app to help me to give up smoking cigarettes. But I'm worried that if I upload it onto my phone it could be used to gather data and other information about me and sell it on - like having a spy on my own phone. So should I be worried, or is the information I'd feed in about my smoking habits and other personal details kept private and not available to third parties for them to use?

A. Recent research has shown mobile health apps are much less likely to share user-data with third parties compared with non-health apps. But many such health apps are designed for tracking the user and their personal behaviour, finding the user's geolocation, and could potentially share this with advert and tracking services without the user's explicit consent. A consumer can disable advert identifiers, adjust app permissions and use advert blockers though, to protect their privacy.

Chapter 2. Empowering you to self-care for yourself or others

Top tips

1. It's a good idea to do a regular health check on yourself- as far as you are able with accessible kit.
2. Get active. If people who are pretty sedentary could be more physically active then that will reduce their chances of developing type 2 diabetes, high blood pressure, heart disease, stroke, cancer and prevent falls. Being more active helps to promote people's confidence too and gives them a purpose and enjoyment each day, as well as preventing their physical decline.
3. Activity trackers and smart watches such as the Apple Watch, Garmin Vivosmart, Google devices and Fitbit offer a range of slim, often waterproof, watch-like bracelets that can monitor someone's heart rate (some relay regularity of their heart rate too), sleep patterns and calories burnt per day with GPS tracking built in. If you've not tried one before, they can really drive you to pursue healthy habits and give you useful feedback.

Preventing your health deteriorating by self-care

It's common for a person to have more than one long-term health condition as they grow older; and some conditions like high blood pressure may not have been diagnosed if there are no symptoms and the person does not receive a regular health check. For instance, cardiovascular diseases such as heart failure, high blood pressure and a heart attack are common in people who have diabetes or are in a pre-diabetic state.

You could buy your own home monitor to take your own blood pressure if you've not been diagnosed as having high levels and it is not checked regularly at clinical reviews. Buy a monitor that's been validated by reliable professionals (check that out at: https://bihsoc.org/bp-monitors/for-home-use/

http://www.bloodpressureuk.org/your-blood-pressure/how-to-lower-your-blood-pressure/monitoring-your-blood-pressure-at-home/);

but don't buy a wrist or finger monitoring device. Make sure the cuff is the right size for your arm (someone who's overweight might need a large cuff size). Taking your blood pressure at home when you're relaxed will give you likely true readings. Keep online records (will be easier to share with a doctor or nurse in future if needs be) of your blood pressure at different times of day – expect it to be lower at night than the morning and to shoot up a bit if you're under stress. Don't get obsessed though. Just check it every month or so unless there's a reason to do it more often. Spotting that your blood pressure is often raised (e.g. higher than 150/80 mmHg) should trigger you to take a diary of your readings to your doctor or practice nurse. The higher it is, the more likely you are to have a heart attack or stroke that could have been avoided if your blood pressure was at normal levels.

It is harder for people to change their lifestyle habits if they are socially disadvantaged or have a low income, are unemployed or in jobs with little control of their situation, and under stress at work or home.
People with an inherently positive outlook (optimists) show greater motivation to self-care for themselves, whereas those with a more negative outlook (more pessimistic) are less motivated to self care.
People with higher motivation tend to perceive their health condition as something that they can gain control over and live with. In contrast, patients with lower motivation take less responsibility for looking after their own health with a degree of helplessness and adopt the attitude that it is the responsibility of others, i.e. the care system or health professionals, to look after them. Elderly patients are less likely to self care because they are often less well informed about their health condition, tend to be more physically impaired and are more likely to take a passive approach to their healthcare, i.e. 'Dr knows best'.
So the emphasis for patients should be on thinking positively, accepting their health condition, building motivation and self-confidence to take more control of their health and wellbeing and live more safely and thus independently, at home.

You need to feel empowered after a clinical review of your health condition with your doctor or nurse – so you should actively engage in discussion with them, tell them what matters to you and what you hope to gain from your consultation, so that you end up with shared decision making about your treatment and care. Make a list of questions you want to ask about your health and wellbeing and remember the information they share with you as you discuss your needs and preferences in respect of the tests, treatment and intervention options they cover. Ask about the risks, benefits and consequences of each option including 'no' treatment or 'no' change to what you're currently doing – but listen and absorb their clinical experience and advice, which should also cover any misconceptions you might have. You can go away and look at reliable patient information about various options online from professional websites or trusted charity sources. Then you should be empowered to make decisions about the care that is right for you at that time (with the options of choosing to have no treatment or not changing what you are currently doing always included).

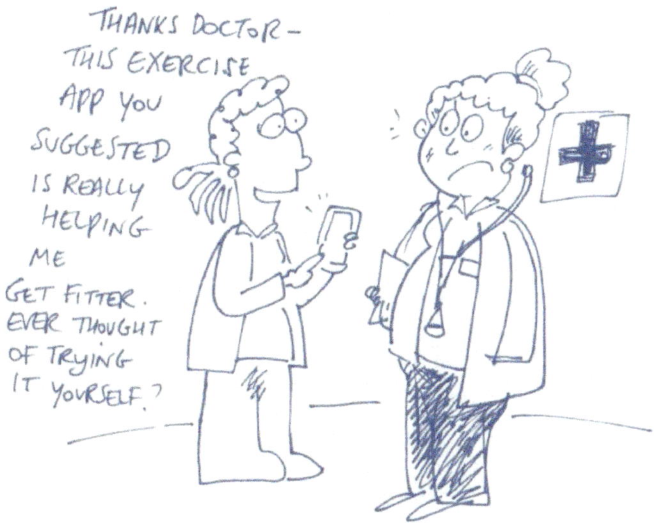
THANKS DOCTOR - THIS EXERCISE APP YOU SUGGESTED IS REALLY HELPING ME GET FITTER. EVER THOUGHT OF TRYING IT YOURSELF?

To improve your lifestyle and sustain that long-term means that you must be interested in changing, then progress to preparing to change, and on to actually making those changes. You may relapse and need encouragement to then repeat the process and maintain the changes you've made.

So take a look and work through the five stages in the cycle of change below to think through what you need to do to overcome any problems in accomplishing your healthy lifestyle goals and stick with your achievements forever.

Five stages of change (e.g. to quit smoking)

1. Pre-contemplation: you've no intention to change your behaviour (e.g. smoking cigarettes) in the foreseeable future.
2. Contemplation: you are aware that a problem exists (e.g. the negative effects on your lungs and circulation from smoking) and are seriously thinking about overcoming it but have not yet made a commitment to take action.
3. Preparation: you are intending to take action in the next few days or months and (may) have unsuccessfully taken action in the past year.
4. Action: you are now modifying your behaviour, experiences, or environment in order to overcome your addiction to smoking. With smoking it's all or nothing. Set a quit date with or without other help (see section below for options). It will take you three weeks to get over the worst of the withdrawal effects.
5. Maintenance: you are working hard so as not to relapse; you're consolidating the gains you've attained by stopping smoking.

Now look at Ben's successful lifestyle changes moving from pre-contemplation to sticking with eating healthy meals and more regular exercise.

Ben's successful lifestyle changes

Pre-contemplation: Ben's mother (aged 74 years) recently had a stroke and was left disabled so Ben and his wife Cath are providing family care. Ben's waist is 44inches and he's recently been told by his practice nurse after an NHS Health Check that he is three stone or so overweight and has a raised blood pressure (hypertension) and is about to start on medication prescribed by his doctor.

Contemplation: Ben considers what weight reduction actions will suit him best – and decides to opt for the 5+2 weekly diet which he's read about in newspapers over the years – eating sensibly for 5 days and then almost fasting for 2 days until he reverts to eating healthily again for the next five days etc., etc. He considers reducing the amount of salt in his meals too and drinking less alcohol.

Preparation: He plans to tackle all his health problems and buys a validated blood pressure testing machine to take his own measurements at home most days which he knows will be more accurate than if he relies on his blood pressure being taken at the doctor's surgery occasionally when he's a bit worked up. Ben signs up to the NHS app to log on to look at his medical records stored at his GP's surgery where he can see that the blood tests he had done after he'd seen his doctor are normal (hurray!). When Ben sees the high blood pressure readings recorded in his medical records he promises himself he'll put this right by shedding much of his excessive weight. And he'll weave in more physical activity by walking to work instead of taking the car which he expects will help his joints and general mobility too. His wife buys him a FitBit watch as a surprise birthday present.

Action: Ben sets his alarm and gets up 30 minutes earlier every day for the first month and does some real exercise – on the exercise bike that's been parked in his garage unused for years or going for a run if the weather's good - well a fast walk anyway. Ben's wife who does all the cooking at home switches to preparing healthy meals with lots of vegetables and little fat or salt – he prefers this for his long-term approach rather than the weekly fasting approach he'd initially considered. He takes home blood pressure readings twice a day for a week after he's been sitting down for a while - to take to his GP for his hypertension review a month later. His GP is delighted to see the listed normal readings which are due to the reliable way Ben has taken them as much as that he's starting to lose weight. When he gets on the scales in the consultation his GP is astounded that he's lost 12 lbs in the last month. He gets home with this good news to find his wife's had a weigh in too and she's lost 7lbs over the last four weeks. Wow!

Maintenance: Ben lost two stones in weight after 6 months, 12% of his former weight! He loves his FitBit - he'd never have bought one for himself, but once he'd learnt what it could do and got used to wearing it, he is forever checking it, which has kept him motivated to get fit and stick with the healthy eating – and he still is only having a couple of pints of beer at the most twice a week when out with friends.

Assistive technology aids to help you look after your everyday health and wellbeing

Medication reminders

If you take a variety of medications in different forms and at various times, it is possible to become confused about what to take and when. This can lead to potentially dangerous situations such as skipping doses or taking too much medication which could cause an exacerbation of your medical conditions or trigger other potential problems such as falling if someone is too drowsy say, from an overdose of medication taken too frequently.

So using pill organisers or blister packs like those illustrated below should help older or confused patients to simplify taking their medication regularly, as prescribed.

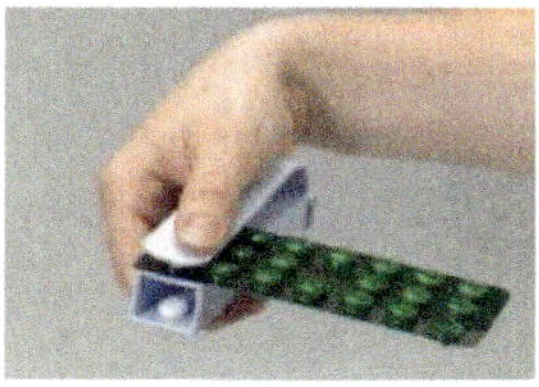

Pill popper: device for removing pills from blister packs.

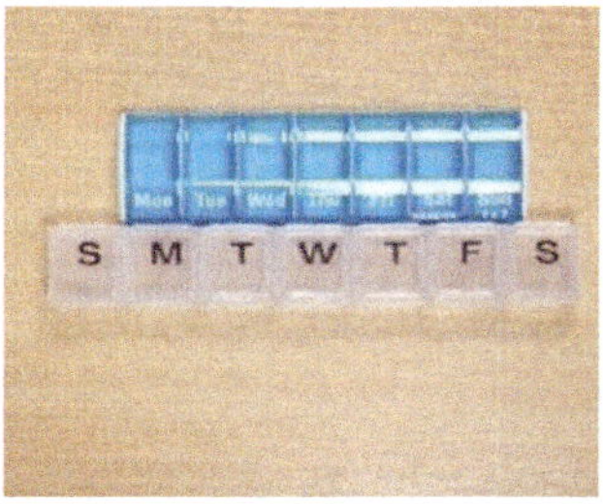

Pill organiser box: 'Dosette' type boxes that you fill yourself, or with assistance from family and carers. These have separate compartments for days of the week and some have compartments with times of day e.g. morning, lunchtime, afternoon and evening. https://www.youtube.com/watch?v=f1FeJ3D1Sg8

Online resources

You can look at a trusted website such as that of Diabetes UK to learn more about a health condition and how to minimise the adverse consequences of the condition. Or watch a video like one on the Asthma UK site as to how others cope with their respiratory condition in healthy ways. Or load a trusted app on your smartphone such as the *Manage Your Health* one highlighted below, to watch the correct way to use an asthma inhaler, or access a personal diary to log symptoms and wellness readings.

Website	Video	App
Diabetes UK	Asthma UK	Manage Your Health
		App Store Play Store

Smart Speaker

You can ask your smart speaker any number of questions. It may not know the answer to all of them but you can certainly gain some usef information from them that could help you to manage your health condition better. Try asking your smart speaker:

- How do I treat diabetes?
- How do I treat knee pain?
- How do I treat asthma?

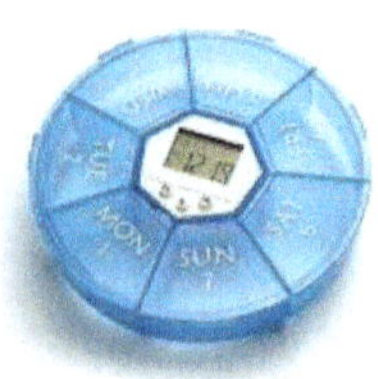

Med-alert pill organiser with alarm: this is a small pill organiser that can easily fit into your pocket or bag and can help you to take your medication on time and at the right intervals. Remembering to do so can be a bit daunting, especially if you have a few different prescriptions to deal with.

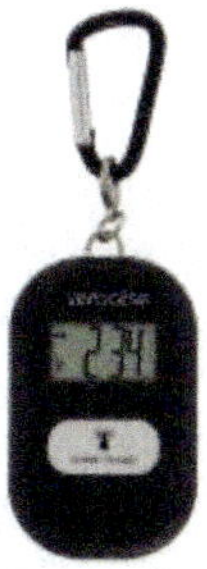

Key chain medication reminder: this handy reminder is useful if you take a lot of medication throughout the day. It has five alarms, which can be set for each time you need to take your medicine.

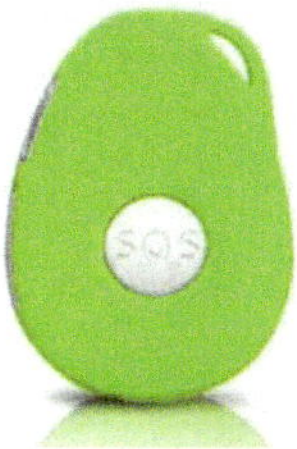

GPS devices: There are many GPS (global positioning system) devices out there, tailored to an individual's needs, to monitor people's whereabouts without being too intrusive and keeping them safe.

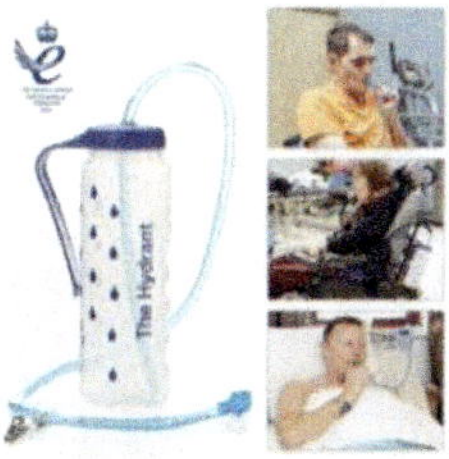

The hydrant drinks system: allows those with limited mobility to take a drink whenever they want, without assistance, reducing the chance of dehydration.

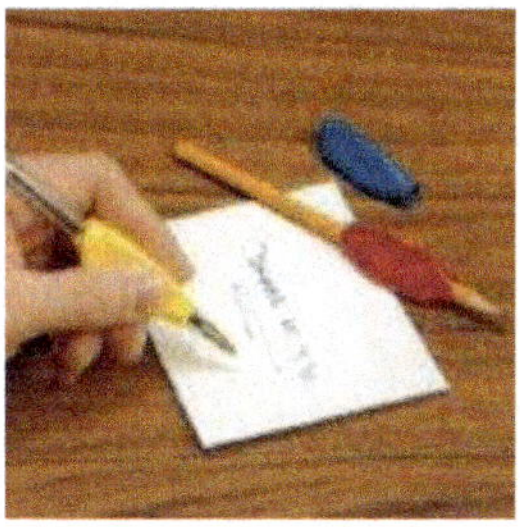

Pen/ pencil holder: Soft and comfortable PVC material provides a more secure grip when placed over pens and pencils. The flexible triangular shaped gripper fits easily over the pen or pencil to assist with stability when writing.

Chapter 3. So quit smoking

Top tips

1. Do your research on reasons why you must give up smoking on the British Lung Foundation website: https://www.blf.org.uk/support-for-you/smoking/why-is-smoking-bad-for-me

   and that of the British Heart Foundation: https://www.bhf.org.uk/informationsupport/risk-factors/smoking
2. Stop now before you damage your health further. Heart disease is common in smokers as is chronic lung disease called chronic obstructive pulmonary disease - COPD. It's common knowledge that smoking causes breathing problems and lung cancer but did you know that people who smoke are up to four times more likely to get heart disease or have a stroke as well as developing other visible effects, such as yellow fingers and teeth, smelly hair and poor eye sight – at a relatively young age too?
3. The NHS Smoke free app can help *you* to stop smoking by providing daily support and motivation. If you stay smoke free for the four week programme you're up to five times more likely to quit for good.

Why quit?

We're talking about your need to STOP smoking - not merely to cut down. So:

- write down the factors in your life that make you want to change. Is it what you will lose otherwise – home, job, family, rows with your partner, money? Is it your health problems that you can see are due to smoking?

- think out how to change your life. This means:
    - being clear about your goal(s)
    - planning and preparing to stop smoking altogether

- not giving up at the first hurdle if you lapse and have a smoke. Most smokers trying to stop make several attempts to quit smoking before they succeed.
- knowing when and how to ask for help (see websites for helpful organisations, or ask your GP or practice nurse).

- soak up support and help from your family and friends in beating your cravings for a cigarette. Be honest about how you are feeling. Talk through pressures and fears that you are covering up.

- try to change your socialising behaviour: avoiding places where you know you'll be tempted or where you used to smoke.

- put the money you're saving by not smoking (e.g. £150 a month) aside and spend it on something great like a holiday.

- be prepared for nicotine withdrawal symptoms: craving to smoke, increased appetite (and so maybe weight gain), restlessness, depression, poor concentration, irritability, disturbed sleep.

- listen to your doctor or nurse telling you to stop smoking. Think about what they've said and the effects on your health (or your family's if you smoke in the house). Research has shown that simple one off advice from a doctor as part of a routine consultation really does help someone to stop smoking.

- adopt a good balanced lifestyle all round with plenty of exercise, a healthy diet, reasonable work/life balance, limited amount of alcohol and no illicit substances. This should help you to pressure yourself to stop smoking and stay quit as an integral part of your good lifestyle.

- Understand the risks to you from smoking- that smokers aged 40 years and under are five times more likely to have a heart attack than someone of a similar age who doesn't smoke. Appreciate that one year after you've stopped smoking, your risk of a heart attack falls to about half that of a smoker; after 10 years from quitting your risk of lung cancer has fallen to about half that of a smoker; and 15 years after stopping smoking your risk of a heart attack falls to a similar level as someone who has never smoked. Whoopee! It is worth persisting.

- try an internet based stop smoking programme e.g. www.quit.org.uk and just do it.

What is the problem?

About a quarter of adults smoke in the UK. Of these two-thirds are likely to say they want to give up. Four-fifths of smokers start when they are teenagers. Passive smoking is bad for people's health too; cot death is more likely in young infants and bronchitis is more likely in children if their parents smoke, as well as it increasing the likelihood that family members and work colleagues develop heart disease or lung cancer. One in two smokers die on average 15 years earlier than those non-smokers in the general population.

How harms happen from smoking

Someone's skin is a bit of a giveaway as to whether they're a smoker or not. Smoking narrows the blood vessels nourishing the skin and their face ends up with broken thread veins. Years of pursing their lips as they draw on cigarettes creates lines around their mouth and eyes and the yellow discoloration of their fingers, teeth and nails is a give away that they're a smoker.

Smoking is the most frequent reason why people die prematurely - from heart and/or lung disease, stroke or cancer primarily. So smoking may increase likelihood of:

- cancer: lungs, bladder, colon, lip, mouth, stomach
- heart and circulation disease: heart attack, stroke, poor circulation especially lower legs and feet, blood clot
- diabetes
- chronic lung disease: obstructive airways disease, worsening of asthma, chest infections
- indigestion, stomach ulcer

- thinning of the bones (osteoporosis) which increases someone's risk of a fracture as their bones are more fragile
- adverse effects on the reproductive system: small baby, early delivery, neonatal death, stillbirth
- psoriasis which is more common in smokers; and improves over the years if they quit
- mental health problems
- poor eye sight: a smoker is more likely to develop age related macular degeneration, making them blind.

What you can do yourself to stop smoking

Benefits start when someone quits. Within three days their taste and smell have improved, breathing's easier and they've more energy. Their risk of a blood clot falls within two weeks of stopping smoking. Three months later their circulation's improved, and after a year smoke-free, their risk of having a heart attack will have dropped to about half that of a smoker. After ten years, their lung cancer risk will be about half that of an ongoing smoker.

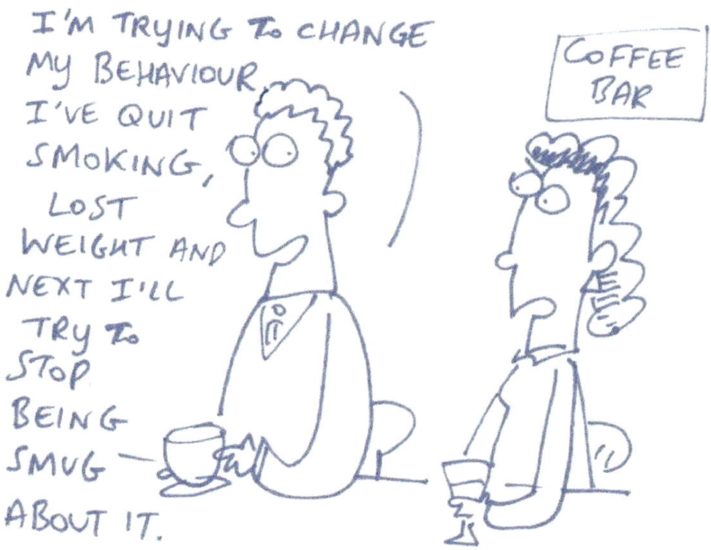
I'M TRYING TO CHANGE MY BEHAVIOUR, I'VE QUIT SMOKING, LOST WEIGHT AND NEXT I'LL TRY TO STOP BEING SMUG ABOUT IT.
COFFEE BAR

Possible treatments to try

Prescribed drugs and other medical approaches

- You could double your chances of quitting by using nicotine replacement therapies – they come as patches, lozenges, inhalers or gum. They reduce your cravings with enough nicotine to ease your withdrawal symptoms. The dose is tailored to match how many cigarettes you have been smoking per day. People usually take nicotine replacement drugs over three months or so, tapering them off gradually. Doctors can prescribe these or you can buy them yourself.
- Prescribed drugs like bupropion or varenicline can help you to stop smoking; research has shown they can double the quit rate. They're not for everyone- not for people who have epilepsy, or women who are pregnant or people who suffer from a psychosis.
- Anti-depressant drugs may be worth trying too, if anxiety and/or depression is all part of your wellbeing problems.
- Trained anti-smoking counsellors can motivate you, and help you to understand the effects of smoking. This can be delivered face to face, or by telephone or text or as one of a group.

Cognitive behavioural therapy (CBT)

CBT helps to reduce someone's psychological symptoms – it can help to get you motivated to improve your lifestyle habits. A *cognitive behaviour programme* might include:

- self-monitoring e.g. keeping a diary of when you crave to smoke again (if you've stopped) or tend to smoke (if you're still smoking)
- stimulus control – developing strategies to reduce your exposure to triggers for lighting up a cigarette
- coping with cravings and high risk situations
- stress management - especially if stress is one of the triggers for you to smoke a cigarette
- relaxation techniques
- learned self-control: breaking the cycle between certain stimuli and smoking
- helping you to build problem solving skills.

Digital aids to help you to quit smoking

Assistive technology

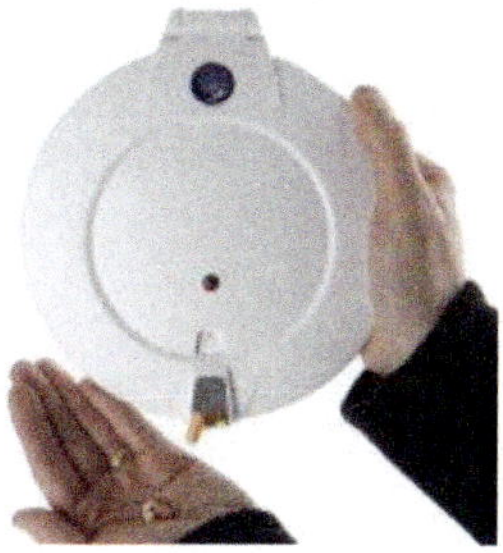

Carousel pill dispenser: help to prompt you to take your stop smoking medication (prescribed by your doctor) where reminders are set up one to two weeks before target date to stop smoking; with agreed frequency; runs for 12 weeks.

Apps

These apps can provide advice and support on stopping smoking:

Look for 'NHS smokefree app' at the App Store or Google Play Store:

Apple

Play Store

Or the app is available at:

https://apps.apple.com/gb/app/smokefree/id687298065

https://play.google.com/store/apps/details?id=com.doh.smokefree&hl=en_GB&gl=US

The Smoke Free app uses over 20 different scientific techniques to help you become *smoke free* by logging cravings, identifying patterns in your smoking behaviour and offering advice.

Look for 'Smoke Free' at the App Store or Google Play Store:

Apple

Play Store

Or the app is available at:
https://apps.apple.com/gb/app/smoke-free-stop-smoking-now/id577767592
https://play.google.com/store/apps/details?id=com.portablepixels.smokefree&hl=en_GB&gl=US

The Quit Genius app uses a combination of cognitive behavioural therapy and a 4-step programme to help you to change your relationship with smoking.

Look for 'The Quit Genius' at the App Store or Google Play Store:

Apple

Play Store

Or the app is available at:
https://apps.apple.com/gb/app/quit-genius-quit-smoking/id1234288038
https://play.google.com/store/apps/details?id=co.digithera.v2.quitgenius&hl=en&gl=US

The My Quit Route app gives you expert advice with scientifically proven tools to help you to quit smoking for good.

Look for 'My Quit Route' at the App Store or Google Play Store:

Apple

Play Store

Or the app is available at:
https://apps.apple.com/gb/app/my-quit-route/id1348024304
https://play.google.com/store/apps/details?id=com.CYS&hl=en_GB&gl=US

The Nicorette Stop Smoking app provides a variety of support tools when you are on the go, including advice, suggestions, and tips to help you tackle every aspect of your path to stopping smoking - from handling your cravings to boosting your motivation.

Look for 'NICORETTE Stop Smoking' at the App Store or Google Play Store:

Apple

Play Store

Or the app is available at:
https://apps.apple.com/gb/app/nicorette-stop-smoking/id1189131363
https://play.google.com/store/apps/details?id=com.jnj.con.synergy

The Stoptober app provides motivation and support to quit smoking and help to track the days someone has been smoke free; it has a savings calculator.

Look for 'Stoptober' at the App Store or Google Play Store:

Apple | Play Store

Or the app is available at:
https://apps.apple.com/gb/app/stoptober/id1034888815
https://play.google.com/store/apps/details?id=com.doh.stoptober2015&hl=en_GB&gl=US

The Manage Your Health app provides information on many health conditions with associated tips and information on diet, quit smoking, alcohol control.

Look for 'Manage Your Health' at the App Store or Google Play Store:

Apple | Play Store

Or the app is available at:
https://apps.apple.com/gb/app/manage-your-health/id1039817165
https://play.google.com/store/apps/details?id=com.keele.vpil

The Craving Coach app is designed for people who have already sought clinical advice and have been advised to quit smoking, improve their diet or reduce their alcohol intake. With 3D videos and images, it provides short 'nudges' that may help you to keep on track.

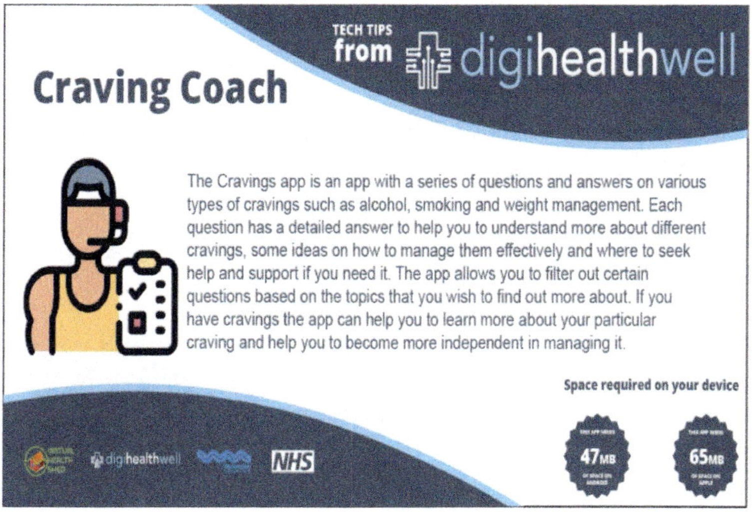

Look for 'Craving Coach' on the App Store or Google Play

Apple

Play Store

Or the app is available at:
https://apps.apple.com/us/app/craving-coach/id1544622157
https://play.google.com/store/apps/details?id=com.vhshed.craving_coach

So here are some key QR codes for you to access for stop smoking advice and support:

Website	Video	App
NHS Quit Smoking	**Eight ways to quit smoking in 2021 LIVE (with Dr Hartmann-Boyce)**	**NHS Smoke Free**

Smart Speaker

These are a great way to utilise technology to encourage and motivate you to stop smoking. Two great features are **lists** and **reminders**. Try using your smart speaker to:

- make a list of reasons why you feel you should stop smoking.
- You can review this list at any time.
- set a reminder for yourself to stay strong and to not smoke. Set yourself a time and add one of the reasons you mentioned in your list.

- ask about the health benefits from stopping smoking.
- ask how to quit smoking.
- listen to relaxing music.
- call a family member or friend. Speaking to a friend or family member can really help to divert you if you are craving a cigarette.

Search term keywords and phrases to find videos or advice that suit your needs:

- tips to beat nicotine addiction
- why should I quit smoking?
- things to take my mind off smoking
- mindful meditation videos to help me to relax and clear my head.

Online information about the risks of smoking and need to quit

Action on smoking and health fact sheets on many topics concerning smoking https://ash.org.uk/fact-sheets/

Self-help advice (NHS) https://www.nhs.uk/live-well/quit-smoking/10-self-help-tips-to-stop-smoking - effects of smoking on the body (NHS)

https://www.nhs.uk/better-health/quit-smoking

Advice on quitting smoking:
www.nhs.uk/oneyou/for-your-body/quit-smoking/personal-quit-plan/

and
www.nhs.uk/smokefree/help-and-advice

Case studies

Hifsa had been smoking for 40 or so years since she was a teenager. She was recently diagnosed with chronic pulmonary obstructive pulmonary disease (COPD) after she'd presented with a recent history of breathlessness when doing simple things like walking upstairs. Her practice nurse gave her a stern warning that she must quit smoking or risk becoming increasingly disabled by her lung function worsening. She'd tried going 'cold turkey' unsuccessfully several times in the past, and nicotine replacement gum hadn't helped much either, but this time she opted for a prescribed drug (varenicline) which has a high quit rate – nine months on she's a non-smoker and has been off any medication for three months now (and is £1,000 richer now she's spending nil on cigarettes – her money tin's full!!).

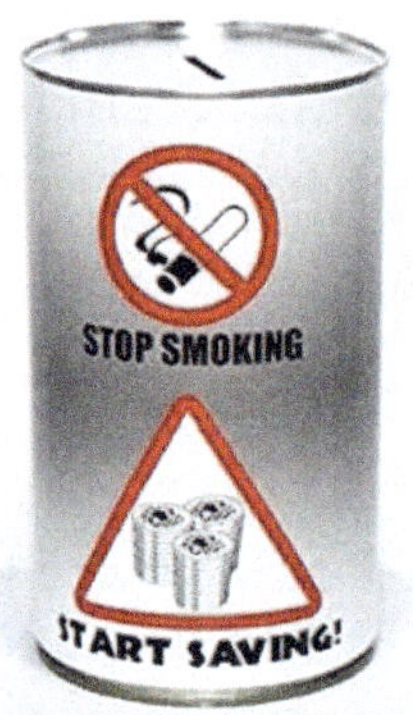

Annie was thrilled to find out she was pregnant - she'd been trying for a baby for 6 months. BUT five weeks after getting that positive pregnancy test she suddenly got tummy pains and started bleeding and had a miscarriage. The nurse explained that she was more likely to have a miscarriage being a smoker....and Annie resolved never to smoke another cigarette. It was a struggle but she was resolute – she would do anything to have a baby- and she wanted the baby to grow healthily in her tummy. So she stopped smoking there and then, using nicotine replacement tablets for a few months to help her beat the cravings to start smoking again. She found that when she stopped smoking food tasted better too. Four years on and Annie has two lovely children aged 1 and 3 years old – and for their sakes and her own, she knows she'll never smoke cigarettes again.

Questions & answers

Q1. Can you tell me where I can get help to stop smoking? I've tried so hard myself and quit several times- but keep starting again.

A. For more information on help to quit where you live search online (e.g. www.smokefree.nhs.uk) for what local services there are near you that offers friendly expert advice, support and encouragement to help smokers to quit for good. Not all local authorities provide free support services though – so find out about the costs and weigh those up – though you're likely to make a financial saving over a short time by quitting smoking! If you need motivation a stop smoking advisor can measure the levels of carbon monoxide (CO) in your body using a monitor. This shows how your CO level drops to the same level as a non-smoker's, just 24 hours after your last cigarette. You should be at least four times more likely to quit smoking with the support of a stop smoking service than if you choose to go it alone!

Q2. How much does the average person save from stopping smoking?

A. Smoking is expensive and you might be surprised at how it all adds up. An average smoker who quits saves around £128 each month, based on today's prices. That's more than £1,500 a year going up in smoke! Use this link to calculate how much you might save yourself:
https://www.nhs.uk/smokefree/why-quit/cost-calculator

Q3. I've tried to stop smoking every New Year for the last five years - but I end up smoking again before the end of January each year. What else can I do?

A. You're only human. The average smoker who gives up makes 4 to 6 attempts first before they do so. Work out why you want to give up - what will motivate you? Is it money saved or that you'll live a healthy life until you're 90+ years old and don't have lung cancer in your sixties? Really focus on those benefits next time you stop smoking. Put cash saved in a box in your sitting room so you can see it pile up. Stick up visual props around your home - you climbing a mountain without getting breathless etc.

Q4. Ruth asked her grandchildren what they thought of adults smoking.

A. Here are some of their personal insights:

1. "I don't want my Nana to smoke – she could die."
2. "It's selfish of parents to smoke as their children breathe it in. If a woman who's pregnant smokes, it damages the baby."
3. "People spend so much money on cigarettes. When my grandad smoked 40 cigarettes a day he spent £000s on packets of cigarettes each year and he could have spent that money on family holidays instead."
4. "Smoking damages your lungs and you won't live as long or be as healthy when you're older."
5. "120,000 people in England die each year from smoking related diseases" (so Morgan found within 30 seconds of searching on Google – the data is there!)

6 "You won't have as many friends if you smoke as a teenager these days – unless they smoke too."
7 "I hold my breath when I walk past my Mum smoking at home – and go upstairs to get away from the smell."
8 "Airports shouldn't sell huge packs of hundreds of cigarettes – it's bad for business if people who buy them die from smoking and stop flying abroad for holidays!"

Adults who smoke need to listen to these messages and use their kids' insights to motivate them to quit.

Chapter 4. So healthy eating it is

Top tips

1. Limiting what you eat boils down to four approaches –

- self-control – a sensible diet and minimal alcohol or sugary drinks
- constraint – stop snacking between meals
- compromise – smaller portions
- substitutes – healthier food with a high fibre content that fills you up for longer or different activities like a new hobby that engrosses you, instead of eating.

2. Everyone's different. You need your own personal approach - find and do whatever works for you to maintain a healthy weight. Do not take good health for granted.

3. It's simple – for someone who is overweight – they must reduce the amount of calories they consume per day (food & drinks) and increase their physical activity in sustainable ways (not as a one off, quick fix!).

Why?

Nearly two-thirds of men and women in the UK are overweight or obese. Numbers are rising year on year. The consequences are not just about people losing their self-esteem or walking slowly as they waddle along - but being more likely to develop some nasty health conditions that they wouldn't have had otherwise if they'd stayed slim, like diabetes or raised blood pressure or heart problems or cancer.

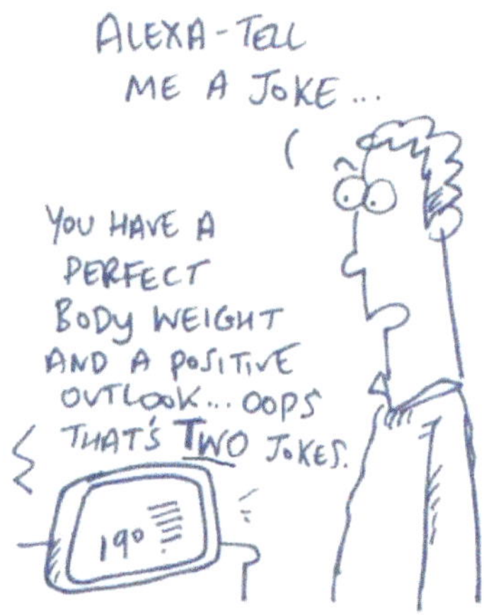
ALEXA - TELL ME A JOKE ...
YOU HAVE A PERFECT BODY WEIGHT AND A POSITIVE OUTLOOK... OOPS THAT'S TWO JOKES.
190

Doctors and nurses have paid a lot of attention to a person's 'body mass index' in the past. This is calculated from the ratio of their weight and height. You can calculate your own body mass index (BMI) by weighing yourself (in kilograms) and dividing your weight by the square of your height given in metres.

Using the BMI as a guide, people have traditionally been classified as:

BMI	
Underweight	less than 18.5
Desirable range	18.5–24.9
Overweight	25.0–29.9
Obese	more than 30.0 (more than 40.0 is known as very severe, or morbid obesity)

You can use your BMI as a general guide as to whether you are at a desirable weight, overweight or obese, but the BMI does not distinguish between the proportion of your body mass being body fat and muscle. Nor does it take account of the distribution of fat around your body. So someone who trains hard in the gym and builds up their muscles may increase their body weight and be classified as overweight or even obese according to their BMI, when in actual fact the proportion of their body fat has shrunk down and they are pretty healthy and fit.

The dangers

On the other hand, someone who might not be defined as obese according to their BMI may have 'central' obesity – a term that has been coined to describe someone with a high level of abdominal obesity. Central abdominal obesity is measured by comparing the circumference of their waist and hips and calculating their waist:hip ratio. This seems to be a good indicator of total body fat. Scientists have found that the relative distribution of fat between waist and hip predicts a person's subsequent coronary artery disease later in life, better than the body mass index does. People with central abdominal obesity are more prone to developing diabetes, heart disease, stroke and some cancers, than people of the same weight and height, whose fat is more evenly distributed around their body. In general, there appear to be increased health risks from obesity when the waist circumference exceeds 94 cms or 37 inches for men, and 80 cms or 32 inches for women.

If you do not exercise frequently, you will find that you gain fatty tissue. This means that your pancreas uses more insulin to break down the fats in your body. Over time the pancreas can wear itself out doing this, especially if it has too much fat to process. This can lead to developing Type 2 diabetes, which then goes on to trigger other health issues too.

Exercise and sticking to a healthy diet aids a person with a health condition such as asthma, to gain better control of symptoms such as shortness of breath – even improving their asthma symptom score by 50%. In another example of how healthy eating helps to control health conditions, acne flare ups are less likely if the person avoids over - indulging in fatty and sugary foods.

If you're overweight and have osteoarthritis affecting your knees and/or hips, then losing weight reduces the mechanical loading effect on your joints – and soon that means you'll have less joint pain and be able to move your joints more easily. Many people accept that they are overweight and inactive but do not make the link between that and the pain in their knees. If your problem is back pain, losing excessive weight around your waist and chest will allow your spine to stay nicely curved, and exercise will help you to recover and be pain-free.

Eating healthily

This isn't just about not gorging on high calorie or fatty foods. It's also about having a balanced diet without excessive fat or carbohydrate, eating fresh food containing lots of vitamins, with a limited amount of salt - less than a teaspoon per day (in any foods or sprinkled on). And of course, the main goal is to balance the amount you eat against how active you are – at work or in your personal life doing household chores, gardening, walking, cycling, sports or other energetic hobbies.

Mindfulness is a good approach to try – so you eat mindfully. That means that you envisage food before it's in front of it, then look at it, next think how you'll enjoy it, then savour each mouthful, appreciate the after taste, then reflect on the flavour and what was great about the food you've just eaten – then start again.

Keep a close eye on what you eat, otherwise you won't realise exactly how much you're eating.

Some overweight people say "I eat hardly anything and yet I never lose weight". Or "It's so small (e.g. a highly calorific snack) it doesn't count"! But you need to focus on exactly what you are choosing to feed into your mouth and take responsibility. You're the only one in control of how heavy your body is and what you look like. If you want to lose weight, that's it, do it – it's only you who can do it – or otherwise, carry on the way you are.

It is difficult to maintain the will power to sustain a long-term change of your eating habits. Many people who successfully retain a reasonable weight have set themselves an upper weight limit – that's their top weight before they make themselves take action to reduce their weight. It's not rocket science.

Either don't eat the food in the first place or work it off so that any excess food is nicely counterbalanced by the energy you expend in doing physical activities – at work or by sport or other hobbies.

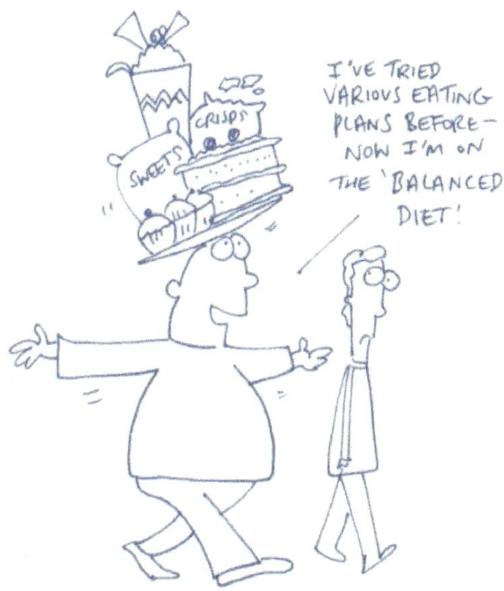
CRISPS
SWEETS
I'VE TRIED VARIOUS EATING PLANS BEFORE – NOW I'M ON THE 'BALANCED DIET'!

Some people make rules for themselves. It might be to never eat any puddings – not ever – not even at Christmas.
Of course, if you don't buy it you can't eat it. So don't keep fattening food in your house on standby.

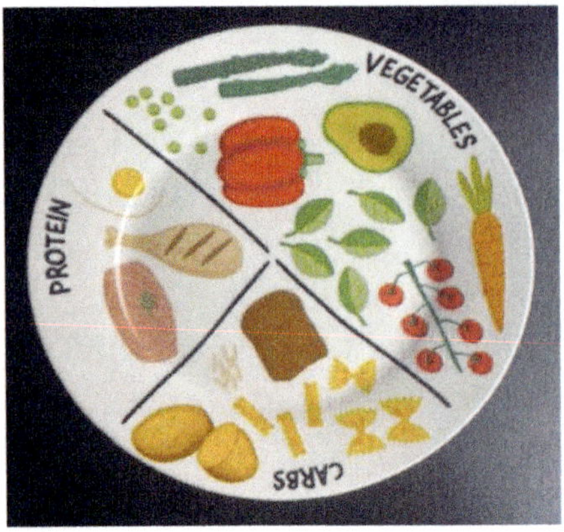

A portion control plate can help you make healthy choices to make sure that you get the right balance of protein, carbohydrates and vegetables and minimal fat in your meals.

Always have a range of low-calorie foods to hand, especially in situations when you know you'll be vulnerable, such as sitting idle on train rides or long car journeys or at the cinema when everyone else around you has popcorn and chocolates. Substitute low calorie food or drink when it makes little difference to you e.g. diet drinks as alternatives when you're out and about, low fat spreads instead of butter, so that you do not consciously feel deprived.

Digital aids to help you eat healthily

Apps and animations

You could download the NHS weight loss guide; a free 12-week diet and exercise plan.

https://www.nhs.uk/live-well/healthy-weight/start-the-nhs-weight-loss-plan/

Look for 'NHS Weight Loss Plan' at the App Store or Google Play Store:

Apple

Play Store

Or the app is available at:

https://apps.apple.com/gb/app/nhs-weight-loss-plan/id1519208548
https://play.google.com/store/apps/details?id=com.nhs.weightloss&hl=en_GB&gl=US

It helps you to create a weight loss plan for the next 12 weeks with weekly challenges in order to:

- achieve safe, steady and sustainable weight loss with a planned daily calorie allowance
- create your own personal weight loss target
- learn to make healthier food choices
- record your progress in losing weight
- make an exercise plan to help you lose weight
- learn how to prevent regaining the weight you've lost.

You can download a chart for each week, stick it somewhere that you can see it such as your fridge, and update it every evening.

Easy Meals is a free app from Public Health England, focusing on healthy foods and meal ideas to help you stay well. It offers over 150 calorie counted recipes.

Look for 'Easy Meals' in the App Store or Google Play Store:

Apple

Play Store

Or the app is available at:
https://apps.apple.com/gb/app/one-you-easy-meals/id1082307333
https://play.google.com/store/apps/details?id=com.PHE.smartrecipes&hl=en_GB&gl=US

A really useful tool to help you to keep track of the amount of sugar you consume in food and drink is the Change4Life Food scanner app, which allows you to scan food and drink labels to check their sugar content. This is a free app from Public Health England that could help you and your family to make a healthy change.

Look for 'Change4Life Smart Recipes' in the App Store or Google Play Store

Apple

Play Store

Or the app is available at:
https://apps.apple.com/gb/app/change4life-be-food-smart/id1182946415
https://play.google.com/store/apps/details?id=com.phe.c4lfoodsmart&hl=en_GB

The Manage Your Health app provides information on many health conditions with associated tips and information on diet, smoking cessation, alcohol control. Look for 'Manage Your Health' at the App Store or Google Play Store:

Apple

Play Store

Or the app is available at:
https://apps.apple.com/gb/app/manage-your-health/id1039817165

https://play.google.com/store/apps/details?id=com.keele.vpil

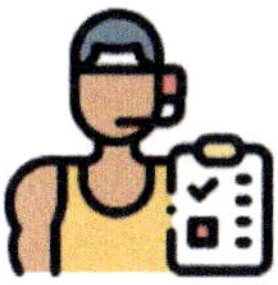

The Craving Coach app is designed for people who have already sought clinical advice and have been advised to quit smoking, improve their diet or reduce their alcohol intake. With 3D videos and images, it provides short 'nudges' that may help you keep on track.

Look for 'Craving Coach' on the App Store or Google Play

Apple

Play Store

Or the app is available at:
https://apps.apple.com/us/app/craving-coach/id1544622157
https://play.google.com/store/apps/details?id=com.vhshed.craving_coach

Websites

You can also visit the NHS website for more tips and advice relating to a healthy diet:

Or https://www.nhs.uk/oneyou/for-your-body/eat-better/

There is an easy-to-use tool to calculate your BMI on the NHS website:
https://www.nhs.uk/live-well/healthy-weight/bmi-calculator

A 30 seconds animation demonstrating the correct method of measuring a person's waist with a tape measure and allowing them to record their waist measurement as part of their health management:
https://extras.bhf.org.uk/patientinfo/waist-measurement_v1.0/app/

The **NHS Better Health website** https://www.nhs.uk/better-health is packed with resources which can help people to lose weight, quit smoking and drinking alcohol, or do more exercise.
It has links to the NHS Weight Loss Plan, or the English Football League who support local fitness and weight loss groups specifically for football fans. It describes, and has links to, seven different weight loss organisations, with their relative costs, as well as some free local authority sessions. Several apps are highlighted, together with links to websites giving nutritional suggestions, activity programmes, diabetes management, and a mental wellbeing plan tailored to your needs, based on answers to a short questionnaire. There is also a link to an eating disorder charity, which has peer support and advice. The 'Get Active' section of the website has video exercise sessions which are free; apps, some of which are free, while others are priced clearly so that you have a wide choice for whatever stage of getting active you are. The links to *Activity Alliance* and *We Are Undefeatable* lead to a wide range of activities, from individualised workouts to activities in groups, both in formal gym settings and using the local countryside, or sports for people who have disabilities.

Quitting smoking, and reducing the amount of alcohol you drink are seen as part of a healthy lifestyle, and are included alongside healthy eating and exercise, with specific apps, videos and links to websites or support organisations.

There are a wealth of recipes, meal ideas and diet plans available for you to use, for free. Here's a few that you could utilise:

Website	Video
NHS Healthy Eating Tips	**The Science of Healthy Eating**

Smart Speaker

Try asking your smart speaker:

- How much fat is there in a particular food item?
- How many calories are there in a particular food item?
- How much sugar is there in a particular drink?
- How do I manage my excess weight?
- Give me ideas on healthy meals I can cook.

Search term keywords and phrases:

- NHS Eat Well
- healthy eating tips
- healthy recipes
- weight loss diet plan
- what are healthy foods?

Case studies

Karen (aged 52 years old) has more or less beaten her diabetes by controlling what she eats. Her advice is "Look at the calorie content of all the food you're tempted to buy and in particular the sugar content." She's changed the type of bread and treats she buys now, lost some weight with eating healthier foods, and her diabetes control is almost perfect – so her GP told her last week. She doesn't need any medication now.

Peter (aged 55 years old): "It's not rocket science. Either don't eat the food in the first place or work it off at work or through regular exercise." Pete has had a personal rule for more than 20 years that he does not eat any puddings – not ever – not even at Christmas time. That means that he can drink the alcohol he wants to and that his normal meals are nicely counterbalanced by the energy he expends in running regularly. If you don't buy it you can't eat it. So don't keep fattening food in your house, and like Pete stop eating when you're full - it's okay to waste food for a good reason.

Anna (aged 28 years old): "When I'm driving in the car, I nibble. So I clean huge packets of carrots and keep them in a pack in the car and at home. If I'm driving back home from work late at night, I allow myself dried fruits and celery. When I'm working late one side of my brain tells me that I need chocolate, whilst the other side says that I don't need it – and I resist the chocolate. I feel much better now that my weight is controlled - more alert and alive."

Questions & answers

Q1. So, if I'm trying hard to lose weight should I just try and eat one main meal a day in the early evening with chicken or fish say, and a maximum of one piece of bread at breakfast and lunch time – and water to drink?

A. Even though you're restricting the food you eat, your diet should be well balanced. So that's at least five portions of fruit or vegetables a day with sufficient calcium to keep your bones strong. It's okay to be hungry during parts of the day. Listen to your body and only eat when you're hungry. Or stop half way through a meal as soon as your hunger is satisfied – you'll eat smaller portions then. Don't leave it too long between meals if going without food makes you feel faint or dizzy. Resist the temptation to eat something to keep you going when waiting for your meal to cook. Eat a low-calorie nibble such as a breadstick or carrot, or do a job or activity that takes your mind off your hunger.

Q2. One of my friends has just been diagnosed with ovarian cancer. The nurse told her that it was more common in very fat women like her! Is that right? Can being overweight cause cancer?

A. Yes being really overweight is regarded as possibly triggering cancer – that someone would not have had if they'd stayed slim. Cancers of the breast, ovary, uterus, prostate, pancreas and colon for instance are thought to be much more likely to happen if someone is obese. Everyone knows that smoking is linked to all kinds of cancers, but the link to being too fat is less well known. Another good reason to keep to a healthy weight throughout your life!

Chapter 5. So quit drinking too much alcohol

Top tips

1. Drink no more than 2 to 3 units of alcohol per day (women) or 3 to 4 units per day (men) (see www.units.nhs.uk/). In the past, weekly limits of alcohol have been suggested as 14 units/week (women) and 21 units/week (men). But the dangers of binge drinking are such that a man taking say 21 units of alcohol on one day of the week can be distinctly harmful.

2. Listen to other people if they tell you that they think you're drinking too much alcohol- they are probably right, and you're in denial.

3. Set your goals - use an online calendar to set yourself targets for restricting how much alcohol you drink each day (and/or other lifestyle goals). They can be small steps, and serve as motivation. You can also share your calendar with a friend or family member who can check up on your goals and offer encouragement.

What is the problem?

It can be difficult to distinguish between binge drinking and alcohol addiction. As many as one third of men and one sixth of women in the UK may be drinking more than these recommended safe limits. And it's thought this might be even more with people turning to alcohol for comfort in the recent pandemic with lockdown restrictions.

It is difficult to give a 'safe' limit to the amount of alcohol an individual person should drink, say per day or per week. Everyone is different – and you cannot lump all age groups together. People change their drinking habits over time. Young people may drink a lot in one go, maybe infrequently; as they get older they tend to drink less at one time but drink more often. All sorts of people have a problem with drinking too much alcohol- it affects all sections of society whatever their age, gender, occupation, ethnicity, social standing etc.

Alcohol gets everywhere in the body and so can cause widescale harm. It can affect for instance your:

- nervous system: dementia, blackouts, fits, hallucinations, disturbed sleep
- heart and circulation: strokes, high blood pressure, enlarged heart (cardiomyopathy), irregular heart beat (maybe temporarily after binge drinking)
- respiratory system: pneumonia
- cancer: liver, oesophagus, larynx, pharynx, breast
- reproductive system: loss of libido, impotence, irregular periods, infertility, foetal alcohol syndrome, unplanned pregnancy
- mental health: low mood, depression, paranoia, suicide
- liver: cirrhosis, cancer, hepatitis, blood vessels burst from your oesophagus (gullet) with pressure effects from enlarged liver
- endocrine system: obesity, overactive thyroid, low blood sugar
- accidents, falls, injuries – and someone with osteoporosis (thinning of bones) is more likely to get a fracture when they fall over.

Lots of research has been undertaken to look at whether drinking regular small amounts of alcohol (especially red wine) does protect your heart. It seems that if there is a benefit, the advantage of drinking a small amount regularly applies only to people at risk of developing heart disease, and only then if they're drinking 1 to 2 units of alcohol per day. Pregnant women are recommended not to drink any alcohol at all, as alcohol can only generate harm, and not give them or their unborn baby any benefits. Women progress to being addicted to alcohol more rapidly than men; they seem to be at higher risk of liver disease, depression etc.

How harm happens

Some people can tolerate huge amounts of alcohol regularly without any harm, whereas others suffer damage to their liver and pancreas and other organs with relatively small amounts of alcohol. Which organ is affected varies with the individual person – the dose of alcohol that damages someone's liver may leave their pancreas unaffected, and vice versa.

A great deal of harm comes from the consequences of alcohol as much as direct effects on your body – traffic accidents involving illegal alcohol levels for instance.

What you can do yourself to cut down alcohol or minimise symptoms

- Complete the FAST questionnaire (see https://www.verywellmind.com/the-fast-alcohol-screening-test). The minimum score is 0 and the maximum score is 16. A score of 3 onwards may indicate hazardous drinking – if so go and discuss your results with your GP.

FAST questions

(1 drink = ½ pint beer or 1 glass wine or 1 single spirits)

1 Men: How often do you have eight or more drinks on one occasion?
Women: How often do you have six or more drinks on one occasion?
never / < monthly / monthly / weekly / daily or almost daily

2 How often during the last year have you been unable to remember what happened the night before because you had been drinking?
never / < monthly / monthly / weekly / daily or almost daily

3 How often during the last year have you failed to do what was normally expected of you because of drinking?
never / < monthly / monthly / weekly / daily or almost daily

4 In the last year has a relative or friend, or a doctor or other health worker been concerned about your drinking or suggested you cut down?
no / yes on one occasion / yes on 2 occasions or more

Scores: for questions one to three – 0, 1, 2, 3, 4 and question four: 0, 2, 4

- Write down the factors in your life that make you want to change. Is it what you will lose otherwise – home, job, family, rows with your partner, money, driving licence? Is it your health problems that you can see are due to drinking too much alcohol?
- Reflect on how to change your life. This means:
    - being clear about your goal(s)
    - spending time in planning and preparation for cutting down or stopping drinking alcohol altogether
    - not giving up at the first hurdle or if you lapse and take a drink
    - knowing when and how to ask for help (see websites for helpful organisations, or ask your GP).
- Soak up support and help from your family and friends in beating your addiction or cravings for alcohol. Be honest about how you are feeling. Talk through pressures and fears that you are covering up by your excessive drinking.
- Try to change your drinking behaviour: how about a few alcohol-free days, never drinking on an empty stomach, going out to socialise later in the evening and returning earlier, thinking of the effects on your body and your family whilst you are actually drinking.
- Cutting back on alcohol should help to prevent attacks of gout if you've suffered from gout before.
- When you have a drink, put the glass down and at a distance away from you, so that you do not drink it unthinkingly.
- Don't accept another drink or allow your current one to be topped up by others unless you actively choose to drink more.

If a doctor or nurse asks you how much alcohol you drink - tell them the truth - you want to be as healthy as possible don't you and get their honest advice?

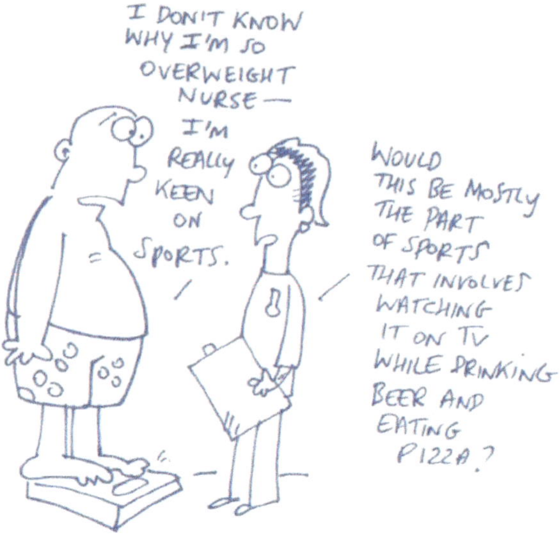
I DON'T KNOW WHY I'M SO OVERWEIGHT NURSE — I'M REALLY KEEN ON SPORTS.
WOULD THIS BE MOSTLY THE PART OF SPORTS THAT INVOLVES WATCHING IT ON TV WHILE DRINKING BEER AND EATING PIZZA?

Possible treatments to try

Prescribed drugs and other medical approaches

- Detoxification in specialist residential setting if severe addiction or have suffered *delerium tremens* in the past when they've come off alcohol, or community settings with daily reviews. Specialist drug regimes help the alcoholic withdraw gradually and damp down symptoms like nausea and vomiting, palpitations, cravings as well as replacing necessary vitamins.
- Antidepressant drugs may be worth trying if anxiety and/or depression is all part of your problems
- People with mental health conditions such as psychoses, like schizophrenia, need urgent help from a psychiatrist specialising in alcohol addiction problems.

Cognitive behavioural therapy (CBT)

CBT helps to reducing psychological symptoms – it probably acts on some of the sources of stress and pressure leading to you developing or coping with your alcohol problem. So use CBT to help you get motivated to change your drinking patterns and behaviour.

A *cognitive behaviour programme* might include:

- self-monitoring e.g. keeping a diary of alcohol consumed
- stimulus control – developing strategies to reduce your exposure to triggers for drinking alcohol- keeping away from pubs for instance!
- coping with cravings and high risk situations
- stress management especially if stress is one of the triggers for you to have a drink
- relaxation techniques
- learned self-control – breaking the cycle between certain stimuli that trigger you into drinking alcohol
- problem solving skills.

Digital aids to help you reduce the amount of alcohol you drink

Online information on the risks of drinking excessive alcohol

Heart UK alcohol guidance

Or look at the link:
https://www.heartuk.org.uk/low-cholesterol-foods/alcohol

NHS Drink Less guidance

Or look at the link:
https://www.nhs.uk/oneyou/for-your-body/drink-less/

Apps

Drink Free Days app - feel healthier, lose weight and save money. Just pick your days to skip alcohol and get practical support to stick with it.

Search for 'One You Drink Free Days' on the App Store or Google Play Store:

Apple

Play Store

Or look at the links:
https://itunes.apple.com/gb/app/one-you-days-off/id1196694906?mt=8
https://play.google.com/store/apps/details?id=com.phe.daysoff

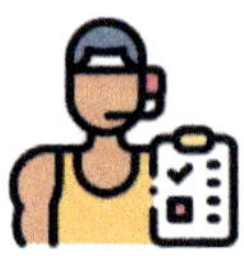

The Craving Coach app is designed for people who have already sought clinical advice and have been advised to quit smoking, improve their diet or reduce their alcohol intake. With 3D videos and images, it provides short 'nudges' that may help you keep on track.

Look for 'Craving Coach' on the App Store or Google Play

Apple

Play Store

Or the app is available at:
https://apps.apple.com/us/app/craving-coach/id1544622157
https://play.google.com/store/apps/details?id=com.vhshed.craving_coach

The Manage your Health app provides information on many health conditions with associated tips and information on diet, smoking cessation, alcohol control.

Look for 'Manage Your Health' at the App Store or Google Play Store:

Apple

Play Store

Or the app is available at:
https://apps.apple.com/gb/app/manage-your-health/id1039817165
https://play.google.com/store/apps/details?id=com.keele.vpil

Website	Video
Cancer Research UK alcohol calculator	**Functioning alcoholics – their stories**

So:

Stay hydrated - Drinking water is a great way to help reduce your alcohol intake. There are many hydration apps available for smartphones and tablets which can remind you when to drink water or other soft drinks to optimise your hydration. Alternatively, smart speakers in your home could be used by using the reminder feature.

Case studies

Alex worked through the five stages of change like Ben did successfully to drop to a healthy weight and exercise regularly (see Chapter 2)

Pre-contemplation: Alex had no intention to change his behaviour – drinking a bottle of wine each night at home when his brother challenged him about how much alcohol he was drinking everyday.

Contemplation: Alex became more aware that his drinking so much alcohol was a problem when he tripped over after drinking four or five glasses of wine on two days running and really hurt his knees both times – no serious damage but that started him thinking about overcoming his dependence on alcohol.

Preparation: Alex planned for cutting down on his drinking – and gave all his spare bottles of wine away to friends and family, reading online about how other people had successfully given up drinking.

Action: Alex opted for 5 days a week without any alcohol- still relaxing with a few drinks in the evening that were alcohol free; and allowing himself one bottle of wine shared across a Friday and Saturday evening.

Maintenance: Alex had only one relapse in the next six months when he went on holiday with a few friends and was drinking at the bar with them. He allowed himself to do that, but otherwise stuck to his plan for 5 days a week free of alcohol, and a moderate amount at the weekend.

Success!

Ann signed up to the Craving Coach app on her Apple watch, as her friend Paula recommended it after they had had a chat about how Ann's excessive drinking was impacting on her work and family life – her teenage children and work colleagues had all confronted Ann about how much she was drinking. The Cravings app had helped Paula to quit smoking last year. Ann loved the visual impact of the 3D videos and images, and the 'nudges' from the app helped her to keep on track, realise how much she had been drinking and switch to an alcohol free month- the goal she set herself.

Questions and answers

Q1. I've struggled to control the amount of wine I drink for sometime. After a heavy day at work I can sit at home on my own and finish a bottle of wine almost every night of the week. I'm not an alcoholic - I just love my wine. How can I cut down?

A. Sounds like you're drinking far too much alcohol. Restock your fridge at home with a range of delicious zero-alcohol drinks, especially alcohol-free wines and beers that you can drink as alternatives to wine.
You've really got to find other ways to relieve your stress from work than by drinking so much alcohol, and solve any mental health issues that you've got. Could you socialise more with friends so you can chat and have a laugh together over coffee or other soft drinks – let them know about how you've cut down on alcohol and maybe update them by Facebook to help you stick to your goal? Could you go out to the gym or go for a run in the evening to have a complete break from work?
You could talk to your line manager and see if the pressures you're experiencing at work can be reduced in some way. Go and see your GP for their advice and talk through any mental health problems.

Q2. Is it true that drinking too much alcohol causes gout? I've some very sore joints in my hand that my GP tells me is gout, and I lied to him that I drank hardly any alcohol (though he might have smelt it on my breath as he didn't look as if he believed me!).

A. Drinking alcohol is widely believed to be one of the causes of gout. It's difficult to state exactly how much alcohol causes gout - but an extra pint of beer or glass of wine regularly might do it. With gout, urate crystals are laid down in vulnerable joints- most commonly the big toe joint but also the ankle, knee, wrist, elbow and finger joints. So control how much alcohol you drink – even cut it out altogether for a few months and see if that improves your gout.

Chapter 6. Stay mobile

Top tips

1. Find exercises that suit you - to get your heart pumping and stretch your back, neck, arms and legs in ways that feel right for you. Just half an hour a day of walking on most days is all it takes for you to help your heart and lungs to be more healthy.
2. Aim for at least 10,000 steps a day. Wear a pedometer or smartwatch that counts how many steps you do. Wear it all day long, when you're walking to work, at work, shopping, gardening or dancing. There are a huge range of cheap and high cost watches and devices; some estimate the energy that you're using to walk those steps as the amount of calories you're burning up, and capture your trends over successive days.
3. Take a look at tips on how to get active from leading health and social care charities and Sport England: https://weareundefeatable.co.uk/

What do you need to do?

Staying physically active and keeping mobile is not just about daily living and maintaining your independence, but also providing you with a good quality of life and alleviating symptoms relating to long term health conditions. So, it is very important that you stay mobile and do not enter a downward spiral of inactivity. Your body strength and maintaining balance are essential. An easy exercise in your own home without the use of any devices is to climb up and down stairs if you can to maintain and promote your mobility. Whether you are completing your household tasks, going for a walk, climbing stairs or riding a bicycle as long as you keep moving, you maintain your health and strengthen your muscles.

Each week you should do at least 150 minutes of exercise that's hard enough to make you breathe more quickly, but you can still talk. That's only an average of 20 minutes a day! If you prefer doing more vigorous exercise, then 75 minutes a week is adequate!

Recent research showed that when older women took light but regular exercise, as for instance going shopping or for a casual walk, they halved their risk of getting a persistent disability compared with women who were pretty sedentary.

Instead of being a couch potato, get out gardening and start growing your own vegetables. Pick a new hobby that you have always dreamt of like dancing or badminton - and make it happen. Find a series of exercises that suit you. Combining exercising and socialising will make the time you spend getting and staying fit more fun, and you'll be likely to stick with it. What about a regular bike ride with a friend or join a line dancing group?

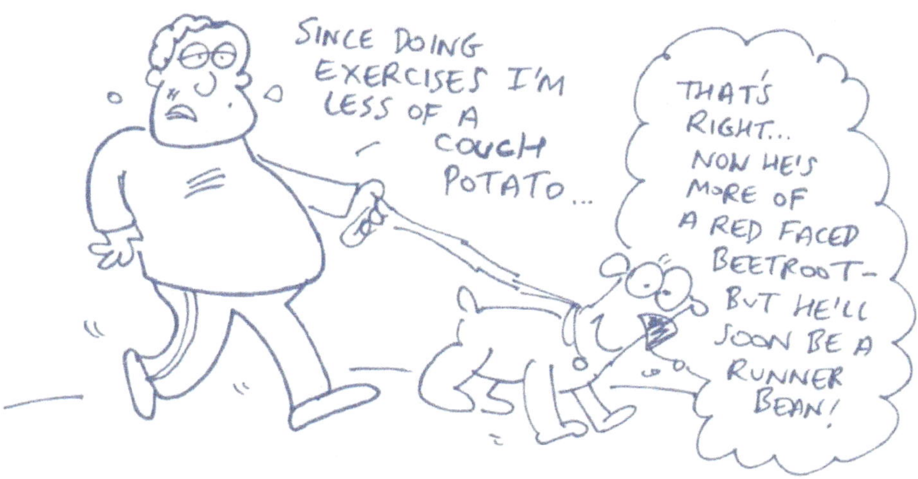
SINCE DOING EXERCISES I'M LESS OF A COUCH POTATO...
THAT'S RIGHT... NOW HE'S MORE OF A RED FACED BEETROOT- BUT HE'LL SOON BE A RUNNER BEAN!

The type of physical activity that you do needs to suit your preferences and circumstances. If you have asthma that is poorly controlled for instance, there may be little point in you attempting a regular two mile walk in all sorts of weather conditions, but you may manage challenging exercise in the warm. If you are someone who is pretty incapacitated from arthritis you might climb your stairs several times in an hour or take a gentle walk to the shops. Activities which fit into your lifestyle and are easily put into action are the most likely to succeed in the long term.

Monitor your heart rate whilst you're active too. In healthy people, the maximum heart rate varies with age, being around 160 beats per minute for a 60-year-old for example. Pitch to achieve 60% of your maximal heart rate for 30 minutes or so, several times a week whilst exercising.

Relieving joint pain

Exercise is helpful for most causes of joint pain, particularly that caused by osteoarthritis. As well as strengthening joints, which helps to relieve pain, it has the additional benefits of assisting with weight loss when required, improving your cardiovascular health (reducing the risk of a heart attack or stroke and reducing blood pressure), elevating mood and improving your quality of life. However, it is not a quick fix solution. It can take weeks to months before you notice a large difference in reducing the pain and improving your functioning – so you need to persevere.

Try a heat and/or a cool pack. Both help joint pains. General approaches for the use of heat and/or cool aids are:

- if muscle spasm and aching is most prominent try a heat pack first. If swelling is prominent try a cool pack. If a pack doesn't work try the alternative pack.
- buy heat (e.g. wheat bags) and cold packs which are widely available, or use items from around the home such as a hot water bottle wrapped in a towel, or bag of peas wrapped in a tea towel. Never place hot water bottles or ice packs directly on your skin though, and only use heat/cold packs for a few minutes at a time to prevent harm.
- warm water which can be very therapeutic; placing your hands in a bowl of warm water may ease pain that's been triggered by movements, and warm showers or baths can help to relieve pain in larger joints.

Pain-relieving medication

All conventional medications have the potential to cause adverse effects. For example, anti-inflammatory medication can cause indigestion, stomach ulcers, bleeding in the gut and kidney problems. So there may be better, safer options to improve your pain such as exercise, a TENS device or using heat and/or ice packs.

Simple paracetamol, anti-inflammatory drugs (e.g. ibuprofen) and co-codamol are commonly used but are not always appropriately. Before you start any medications, first consult with your pharmacist or GP to check that they are a safe option for you. General advice about the use of pain-relieving medication include:

- start with topical medications (i.e. anti-inflammatory rubs and/or creams) particularly for hand and knee pain.
- paracetamol is usually safer than an anti-inflammatory tablet or capsule.

Tips for boosting physical activity for people who are overweight

1. Build up slowly towards 30 minutes of moderate intensity activity a day. The 30 minutes can be accumulated throughout the day in 10-15 minute bouts. Moderate intensity means breathing slightly harder than normal but still within the 'comfort zone' whereby the activity can be done whilst talking at the same time.

2. To achieve optimal weight loss, consider extending some sessions to 45 minutes or more as this will encourage the use of fat as an energy source.

3. Increase the amount of daily routine activity such as gardening, shopping, housework, walking and so on.

4. Decrease the amount of time spent in sedentary activities and try not to sit down for more than 30 minutes at a time.

5. The best activities for weight loss are those involving large muscle groups, which are anaerobic in nature, such as walking, swimming or cycling.

6. Consider weight-bearing exercises such as walking and climbing stairs as they help to conserve muscle mass, and maintain strength and resting metabolic rate.

7. Find physical activities which you enjoy.

The table below describes the average number of calories per hour used up by the varying activities included here, and illustrates the differences between the way men and women function.

Average hourly calories used up during various physical activities (the actual calories used up by an individual will depend on their age, height, weight, speed and strength)		
Activity	**Women**	**Men**
Bowling	207	270
Cycling: moderate	192	256
hard	507	660
Ballroom dancing	264	352
Driving a car	108	144
Active gardening	276	368
Golf	144	192
Ironing	120	160
Walking: moderate	168	224
Running: moderate	444	592
hard	692	900
Sitting: at rest	84	112
Skiing	461	600
Squash	461	600
Swimming: moderate	230	300
hard	480	640
Table tennis	300	400
Tennis	336	448

Staying safe at home: four stages in risk management to help someone to stay safe:

- identify key risks and any triggers and previous adverse events.
- analyse each risk- how common is it, are there patterns or trends, what impact does it have, does that impact matter?
- control the risk – what can be done about it? E.g. buy safety technology and other products, and implement changes in the home as necessary.

- cost the risk – look at the cost of getting it right versus the cost of a risky outcome.

Sometimes managing or controlling one risk has the knock-on effect of creating new or greater risks elsewhere. If you do not have a grasp of the bigger picture, you can make things worse – and more risky.

Digital aids to help you to stay mobile

Apps

You may feel you need motivation when it comes to being and staying active. Some apps help you to keep track of the exercise that you do.

Active 10 is an app created by Public Health England that helps you to set goals, track your daily steps, and motivate you to set and achieve your targets. The 'One You Active 10 Walking Tracker' app is available to download at:

Apple

Play Store

Or the app is available at:
https://apps.apple.com/gb/app/one-you-active-10-walking-tracker/id1204295312
https://play.google.com/store/apps/details?id=uk.ac.shef.oak.pheactiveten

The EXi app offers a tailored exercise plan by creating a 12-week exercise plan based on health information entered by the user. The plan includes tips, advice and guidance on how to keep or get active in and around the home; it then sets the duration and intensity of the exercise based on this information: https://www.nhs.uk/apps-library/exi/

Find the 'EXi – Exercise Prescription' app at:

Apple　　　　Play Store

Or the app is available at:
https://apps.apple.com/gb/app/exi-exercise-prescription/id1156093317
https://play.google.com/store/apps/details?id=com.iprescribeexercise.app.android.iPrescribe

Couch to 5K - Get off the couch and running 5K in just nine weeks. Grab your trainers and follow the step-by-step audio instructions of the 'One You Couch to 5K' app:

Apple　　　　Play Store

Downloads of Couch to 5K, surpassed five million by July 2021. The app was downloaded 2.36 million times since the pandemic started (March 2020 to July 2021) by people seeking to get more active during lockdown. Couch to 5K is a free running plan for beginners provided by Public Health England (PHE) and the BBC, helping those who don't regularly exercise or keep active to take positive steps to boost their own health and fitness. Regular running has been shown to reduce the risk of long-term illnesses, such as heart disease, Type 2 diabetes and stroke, as well as helping you to maintain a healthier weight and improve your mood. Designed for people who have done little or no running, the app provides a guided commentary from a celebrity coach and helps users to easily track their progress by doing at least three runs per week.

Or the app is available at:

https://itunes.apple.com/gb/app/one-you-couch-to-5k/id1082307672?mt=8
https://play.google.com/store/apps/details?id=com.phe.couchto5K

For tips, advice and guidance on how to keep or get active in and around your home from Sport England, take a look at: https://weareundefeatable.co.uk/

Using assistive technology to maintain your wellbeing and independence

There are many assistive devices and technology that help someone to stay mobile. These range from non-electronic simple products such as walking sticks to easy to use electronic devices such as GPS trackers. These systems support an individual to maintain their wellbeing and independence along with safety.

Walking stick A walking stick or a cane is a fantastic companion to support you to keep moving. Although there are several options, most individuals benefit from a stick that has a single tip. There are quad tipped sticks, which are normally used by individuals who are recovering from a clinical episode such as a

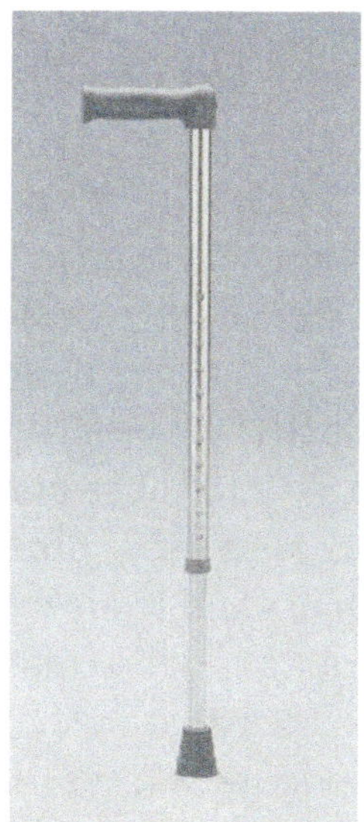

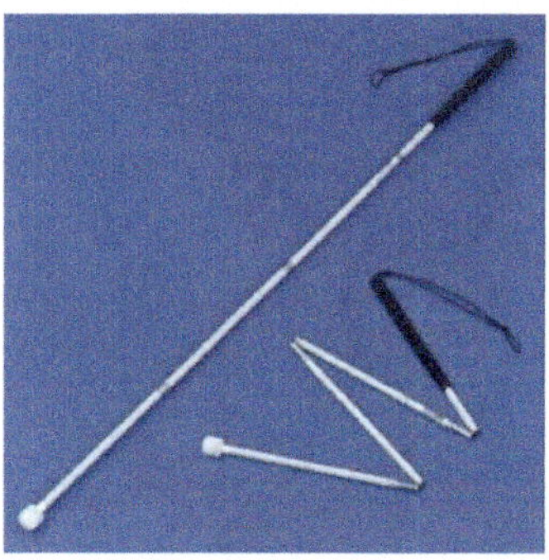

stroke. You need to make sure that you can maintain a good posture whilst using this stick. This relates to the length of the stick and the shape and size of the handle.

As a good measure, the handle of the stick should come up to about your wrist when the stick is positioned on the floor. Make sure you choose a type of grip that is comfortable for you. Sometimes a custom-made grip made of foam that's shaped to fit your hand will work well.

Walker (or walking frame)

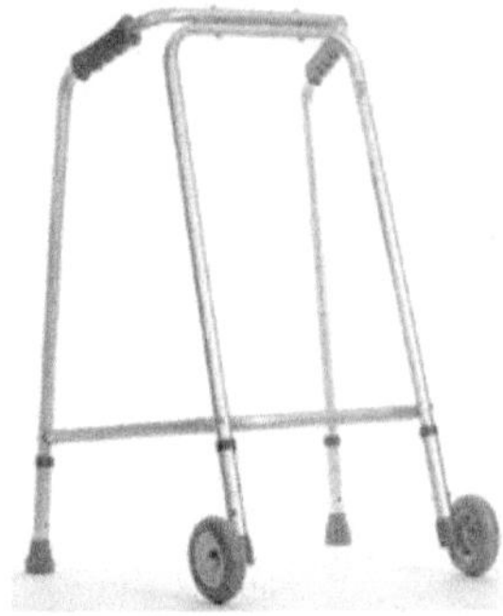

Some people prefer, and feel comfortable with, a walker. Walkers are sturdier than walking sticks and they come in varying types and sizes. A commonly used walker has four rubber-tipped legs that you pick up to move. Walking frames are designed to offer additional support to the user and come in many different sizes and designs, but also can come with many additional features, such as wheels so they are easier to push, trays, so that items can be carried. Some have two wheels on the front legs which is helpful for weight-bearing activities. On the other hand, a three-wheel walker is easy to manoeuvre whilst providing good balance support. The four-wheel walkers are great for those who do need to rely on their walker for help with their balance. Walkers come with appropriate grips; most are plastic but sometimes a foam grip can be more beneficial.

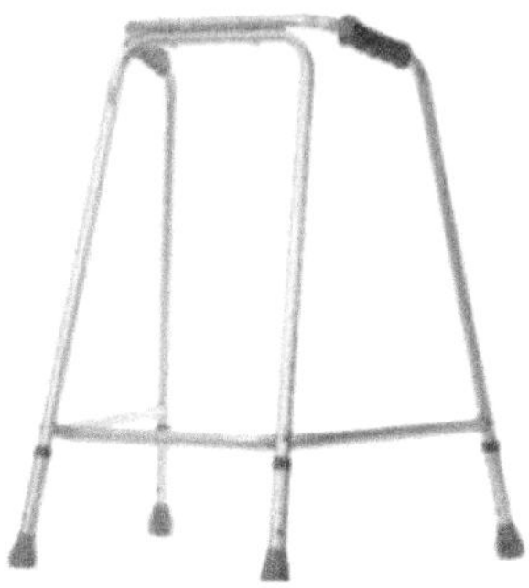

Wheelchairs and scooters

Wheelchairs and scooters provide the next level of mobility. In terms of wheelchairs – there are two types: manual and electric. Self-propelling, manual chairs need the user to have good upper body strength. However, electric wheelchairs can support individuals who have compromised body strength; these are battery-powered and depending on where the motor is based they come in different types: rear-wheel drives, mid-wheel drive chairs and front-wheel drive chairs. You can choose them, depending on your needs for manoeuvrability. A scooter can take you from place to place with a push of a button. These are ideal for individuals who can sit upright for a reasonable time but can't walk long distances. The choice of scooter depends on whether you want to use this mainly indoors or outdoors.

Fitness tracker

Over the years, individuals have used various forms of trackers including simple step counters or pedometers. With the advances in technology and the use of smartphone and its applications, fitness tracking has become simple. A fitness tracker is a device that tracks your movements, similar to a traditional pedometer, a wearable device or a smartphone app.

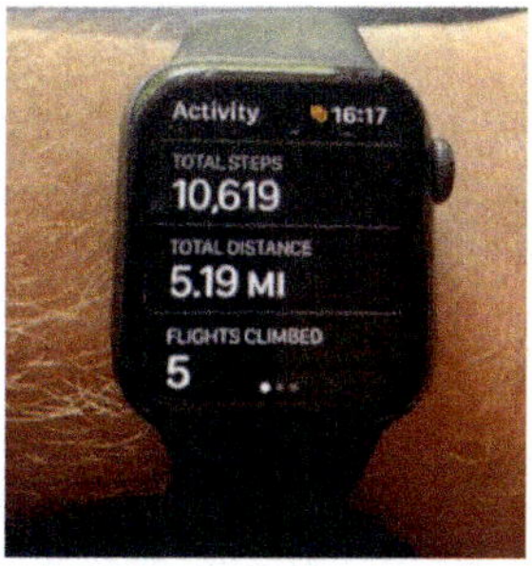

These trackers can remind you periodically that you need to get active and help you to increase your daily step count. One of the other advantages of using fitness trackers is their capability to visualise how long you have been active, how many steps you have taken and how many calories you have burned that day. Seeing this progress helps you to set goals and keeps your motivation up to achieve your physical activity goals over time.

Website	Video	App	
British Heart Foundation site	**Beginners’ stretching exercises for general flexibility**	**HASfit**	
		Apple	**Play store**

Smart Speaker

Smart speakers with a screen such as the Echo Show have a built in web browser and can access the internet, and therefore any information on webpages as well as videos on sites such as YouTube. You can also use smart speakers to interact with additional smart technologies, such as plugs sockets, light bulbs, and central heating thermostats. These are incredibly useful, especially for those with mobility challenges. Try search term keywords and phrases:

- morning stretching routines
- chair exercises
- fitness tracker
- balance exercises
- exercise as you get older
- Couch to 5k

Case studies

Rob had heart surgery 14 years ago when he had an aortic valve replacement. He feels as fit now in his early 70s as he did in his 40s. He puts that down to lots of regular exercise, walking the dog several times a day and opting for a healthy diet. He says another reason he feels so well is that now he's retired he's his own boss rather than when he was working in the building industry and being ordered to travel to different sites and do challenging jobs with too little support. He never smoked cigarettes, but used to have friends who did- they've died now!

Emma has learnt Tai Chi exercises which have been shown to prevent falls in various research studies. Tai Chi combines deep breathing and relaxation with flowing movements as part of the physical activity that improves people's balance and coordination. Emma joined a weekly group at her local community centre, but she continued exercising with them by a video-link during the pandemic on a regular basis.

Questions and answers

Q1. Since I got a fitness tracker watch for my 60th birthday from my family I've gone berserk trying to run five miles a day, several times a week with my son. Sometimes this gives me chest pain - probably my muscles groaning. Should I keep going to be more healthy or is this a sign of pushing myself too hard?

A. Self-monitoring devices like your smartwatch can have unforeseen consequences like encouraging overly-competitive urges like you describe – racing too fast to reach extreme exercise goals. That might induce a heart attack in someone pushing themselves too hard and that would definitely be unhealthy. Consult your GP about your chest pain in case it's angina - and put your new watch in a drawer until you've had the all clear.

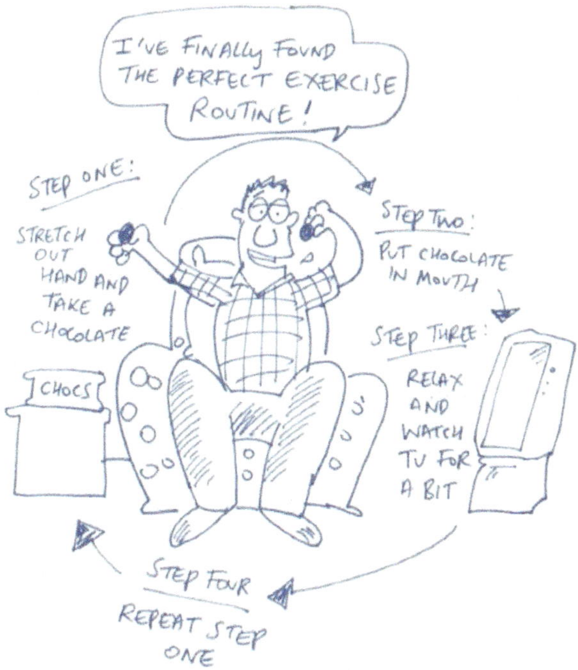

Q2. I sprained my ankle a couple of years ago after tripping over and it's hurt ever since if I go for a run, so I'm sitting in a chair most days. Should I be exercising more?

A. Exercise can increase your pain transiently. This does not necessarily mean that you must stop exercising. As a general rule of thumb, if your pain has not dropped to its usual level after two hours, next time reduce the amount of time you that you exercise for, or the effort that you put in, and build up your fitness more slowly.

Chapter 7. Overcoming frailty and poor balance

Top tips

1. People who do too little activity will get thinner bones. Regular exercise will improve your balance and muscle strength. The best type of activity is one that physically stresses the bone, such as jumping, running and skipping. That will increase bone density in teenagers, maintain it in younger adults and slow its decline in older age.
2. Home based exercise can help you to build your muscle strength (in your legs, feet, body, arms) and balance, and prevent you from having falls.
3. It's worth checking with your doctor or pharmacist that any medication that you take is not making you too drowsy (and so more like to trip up and fall); and if so, if they can try switching you to an alternative treatment that your doctor thinks will be likely to work just as well.

So what is frailty?

Frailty is the gradual loss of inner reserve as someone grows older. It's more likely to be described in people's everyday conversation as 'slowing down', or 'more of a struggle' or 'things take longer'. The more that you boost your bodily strength and mental resilience, the better you manage the threat of frailty to your health and wellbeing and stop it progressing so that you are then less likely to experience an acute illness, or a fall, or worsening immobility.

Lots of people do fall over as they get older, as they become increasingly frail and more likely to trip up. And with weakened bones as they age, they are more likely to end up with a fracture. It's estimated that one third of people older than 65 years old and half of those aged 80 years or older have a substantive fall at least once a year and that adds up to over three million falls annually in the UK by those aged 65 years or older. Falls are the most common cause of death from injury in people who are over 65 years old!

Balance and gait impairment are core features of frailty, and key factors in someone's risk of falls. Frailty cannot be cured, but it can be controlled, or at least its progression slowed down by redressing unhealthy lifestyle habits, preventing falls, and boosting someone's mental wellbeing such as through social interactions.

Osteoporosis is the term that doctors use to describe the gradual thinning of the bones, or officially 'degenerative bone disease'. Osteoporosis usually occurs in elderly people, or in younger people who have other reasons for it, such as taking steroid or thyroid drugs. Women who have an early menopause are more likely to get osteoporosis. It runs in families too. The low bone mass and low mineral density means that your bones are more brittle and more prone to fracture. Your bone density gets less as you get older, whoever you are. Unfortunately when someone with osteoporosis falls over, they are more likely to break their bones which have become thinner. People don't necessarily realise that their bones are weak and they're at risk of a fracture, as osteoporosis is painless. But sometimes people are left in pain after a fracture, depending on where it is sited.

The most common bones to be fractured after a minor trip or fall in someone with osteoporosis is their hip, wrist and spinal bones. So such a fracture should be a clue for doctors treating them to investigate if they have osteoporosis, by testing their blood and bone density with a specialised scan. You can prevent osteoporosis to some extent – so don't be bone idle! Take regular weight bearing exercise and go for a diet that's rich in calcium and vitamin D; that's milk, cheese and other dairy foods and tinned fish particularly. Sunlight boosts vitamin D levels. Avoid smoking or drinking lots of alcohol; if you smoke or are a heavy drinker you know what you should do – STOP!!

It doesn't pay to be thin when you're considering how to prevent osteoporosis. So a reasonable body weight for your height is what you should be aiming for, to put your hips and legs under reasonable stress. Anorexia is a real threat to maintaining bone density.

If you've got osteoporosis, the last thing you want to do is to fall over and risk a fracture. Check that your home and work environments are safe.

Improve your lighting, remove rugs or other hazards lying on the floor to make it less likely that you trip over.

Focus on your feet

Custom made insoles or orthoses may help by reducing pain when fitted in someone's shoes who suffers from plantar fasciitis. It's important to have correctly fitting footwear including socks.

Including a gel innersole inside each shoe can help to prevent ulcer and callous formation by reducing the impact of your foot striking the floor when you're walking or running.

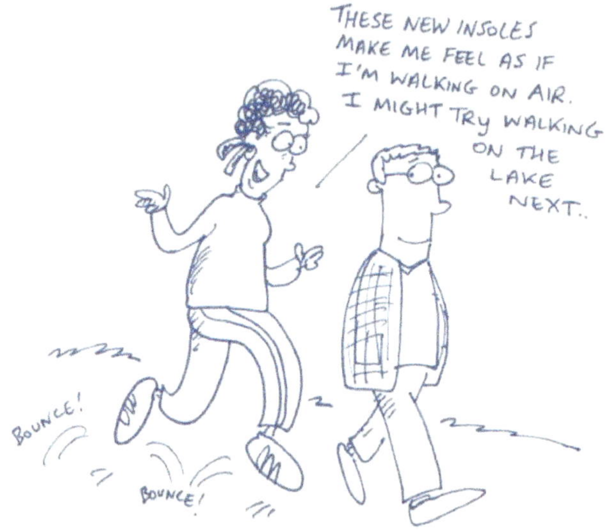
THESE NEW INSOLES MAKE ME FEEL AS IF I'M WALKING ON AIR. I MIGHT TRY WALKING ON THE LAKE NEXT..
BOUNCE!
BOUNCE!

Check your feet daily – use a mirror to look underneath both of your feet, at your soles. Look out for any cuts, grazes, swelling, changes in colour of skin or nails and changes in the shape of your foot too.

Take care cutting your nails; if you struggle get someone else to cut them and if you are suffering from a loss in sensation it may be worth seeing a podiatrist for their view and advice. Buy sensible shoes that are well fitted, with velcro straps or elastic laces if you find typing knots in laces difficult.

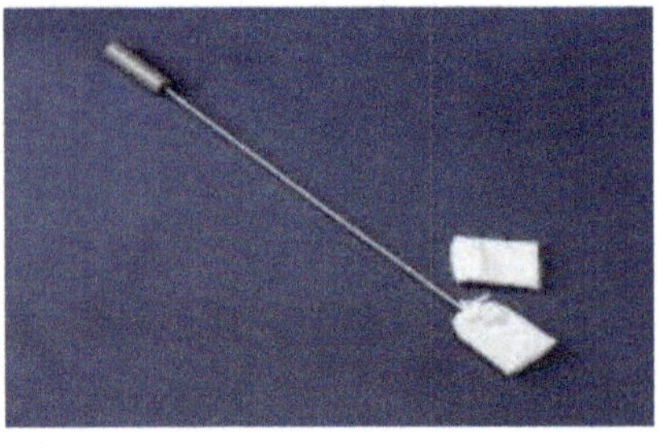

Long handled toe cleaner-
The toe cleaner can help you clean your toes with bending too much and can also aid with cream application.

Digital aids to help you to overcome your frailty and improve your balance

Exercise videos

The range of videos below have been prepared by the cardiac (heart) rehabilitation team of University Hospital North Midlands. Try the exercises shown in these videos to help you to keep fit and get your joints more supple. They should also help people with heart or lung conditions or those who've had a heart attack or need to get their strength back after a nasty illness or operation.

Take a look at the following video to help you rate your perceived exertion before starting the exercises to help you know when you have 'had enough' and it is time to stop:

Or look at: https://www.youtube.com/watch?v=90dJgldll2Y&t=1s

These '**balance and posture'** exercises are particularly useful if you have had a stroke or a chronic neurological condition such as multiple sclerosis (MS) or simply to help you as you get older and find that your balance and coordination is not as good as it used to be.

Good balance is needed for lots of day to day activities, such as walking, climbing the stairs, housework and DIY activities. Maintaining good balance and posture can have lots of benefits to your overall health and wellbeing too. It can reduce your chance of injury, joint and muscular pain and can help to reduce your risk of falls. Guarding against these things is particularly important as you age. This series of videos guides you through three gentle home exercise sessions without any equipment, to help you to improve your balance, posture and coordination. They are also suitable to complete if you have long-term health conditions such as heart or lung conditions.

After you've tried out the 'balance and posture' videos and feel comfortable completing them, you can move onto the '**coordination**' video which demonstrates some more advances exercises that you can try:

1. Balance exercise: take a look:

or:
https://www.youtube.com/watch?v=niovkkFlD4s

2. Posture exercise: take a look:

or:
https://www.youtube.com/watch?v=mXtzXdxxb2c

3. Coordination exercise: take a look:

or:
https://www.youtube.com/watch?v=z6Vw4knQjKI

The **seated home exercises** are a series of six exercise videos that can be done within your home. All the exercises can be completed whilst sitting in a chair; your dining chair is a good choice to help you to sit upright and offer you support. These workouts are a great and safe option for those who have problems with their balance and are keen to improve their fitness and stay active at home. You should be able to complete these exercises if you have long-term health conditions and they can help you to keep active and independent too.

Choose the ones where you feel comfortable with the length of time and intensity, and progress through the whole series of six as your strength and fitness improves:

or look at:
https://www.youtube.com/playlist?list=PLkNJgnY2UkGAMU5o7ZtUHgchOVA_Zo7TO

Next the six **standing home exercise** series of videos with increasing length of time and intensity that can be done within your home, making use of everyday household items to develop your workout. They are completed in a standing position. (So if you have problems with your balance take care and stick with seated exercises if you feel too wobbly doing exercises standing up). All these exercises are suitable if you have a heart condition and/or other long-term health conditions to help keep you active and independent. They vary between a 10 minutes to a 30 minutes exercise session, each with an appropriate warm up and cool down period.

or look at:

https://www.youtube.com/playlist?list=PLkNJgnY2UkGBFbMu5R6cdA49cu01QAz7F

Assistive technology that may help

Footwear choice contributes to maintaining good balance. There is a plethora of research that has looked at the relationship between footwear and balance resulting in falls or fear of falling. Various footwear characteristics, including shape and materials of upper, sole hardness and tread contributes to someone's balance. Research studies have shown that insoles with tactile surfaces help to improve balance.

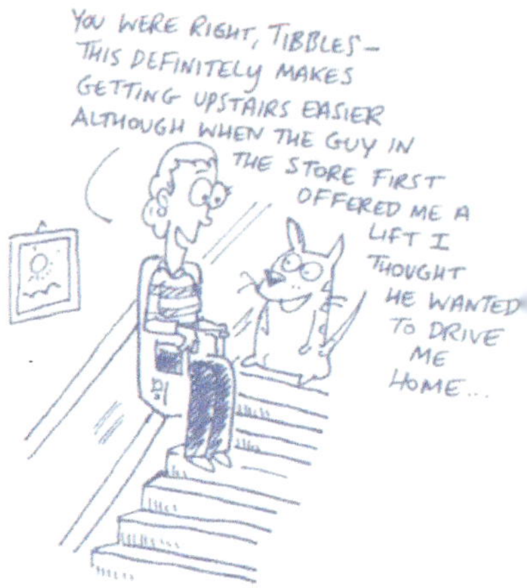
YOU WERE RIGHT, TIBBLES – THIS DEFINITELY MAKES GETTING UPSTAIRS EASIER ALTHOUGH WHEN THE GUY IN THE STORE FIRST OFFERED ME A LIFT I THOUGHT HE WANTED TO DRIVE ME HOME...

GPS devices

Personal alarms and a variety of GPS devices are commonly used to allow people to call for assistance if they have an accident or a fall. This feeling of safety helps an individual to remain independent for longer. Also, these devices offer peace of mind to the family.

A simple GPS based tracker helps to locate older people in case of an emergency or if they get lost. It offers much-wanted independence to individuals, whilst the family can still locate them anytime simply, for example, via an application on their mobile phones. This undoubtedly minimises unwanted stress for the family. Some of these GPS trackers also have personal alarms that are simple to use. They normally feature one big button that can be pressed to get help quickly if the individual faces difficulties.

Safety buttons

These personal protection devices are small devices that allow individuals to discreetly press a button to signal to family and friends that they are facing a difficult situation, particularly when they can't use their phone or call for help in other ways. These devices use Bluetooth technology to talk to a smartphone. This smartphone will have an application that tracks GPS data and sends a warning message to a list of contacts.

These devices offer multiple alerts which have varying meanings. For example – a press of a button could say "I have arrived" or it could send a message to warn someone of a potential accident or it could send an 'SOS' seeking immediate help.

In both cases, a commercial solution provider might offer a wide variety of services based on one-off payment of a subscription. You must choose the right technology with the right level of service.

The Handi SOS has a bluetooth safety button which pairs to your phone. When pressed, it sends alert SOS text messages and your Google Maps' location to selected contacts. There are no subscriptions and no monthly fees.

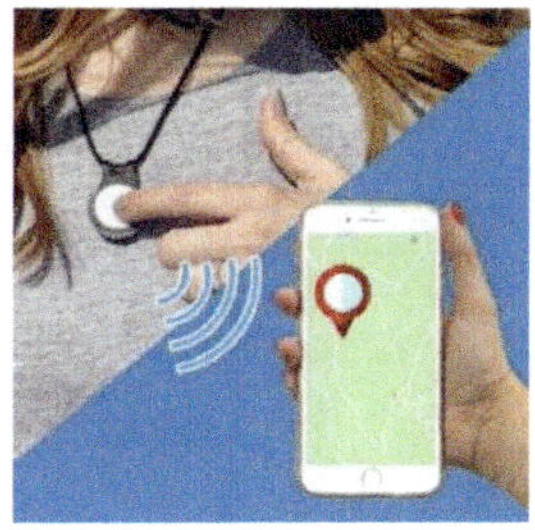

https://www.handisos.co.uk/product/handi-sos-ios/

Website	Video	App
A practical guide to healthy ageing	**Simple ways to help with medication**	**Keep On Keep UP** Only available in Apple App Store

Smart Speaker

Being voice activated, smart speakers can offer ease of access and allow interaction only by asking. This can become very useful should you live alone, have a fall and need to call for help. You can also integrate plug sockets, light bulbs, central heating thermostats, security cameras, and even a kettle. These are incredibly useful for those with mobility challenges. Chair yoga is a gentle form of yoga that is practised sitting on a chair, or standing using a chair for support.

Search term keywords and phrases:

- Fall prevention
- Frailty risk identification
- Strength exercises
- Balance exercises

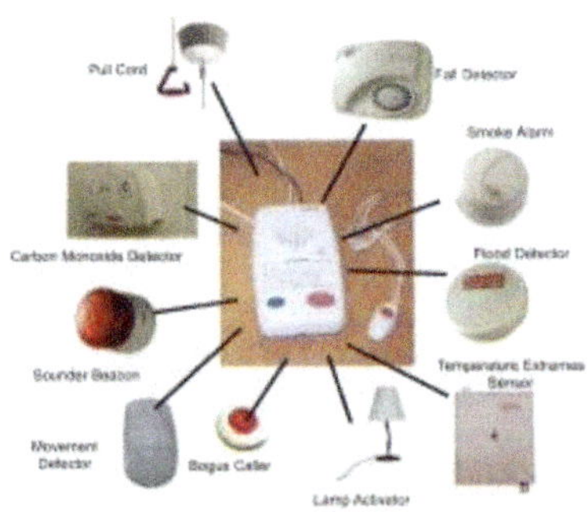

Telecare equipment Telecare devices are designed to call for help if someone has a fall or needs support whilst at home in an emergency. The types of devices that can link up to the care call system consist of fall detectors, smoke detectors, flood detectors, carbon monoxide detectors, movement sensors, door sensors, temperature sensors and light activators.

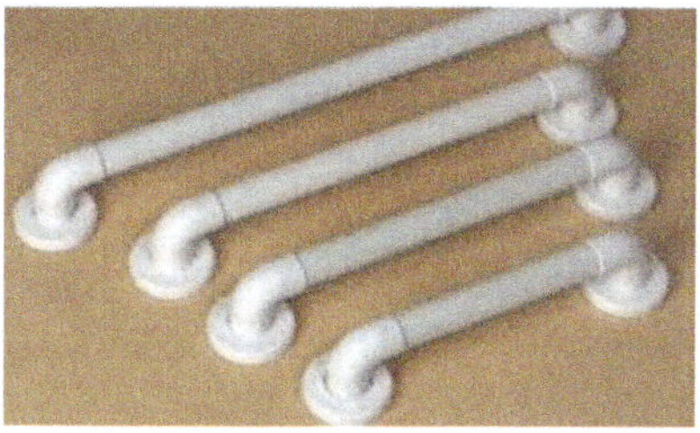

Grabrails Grabrails can help with many different tasks around the home, should you find yourself struggling to get in and out of your property, or if you are struggling to get on and off your toilet.

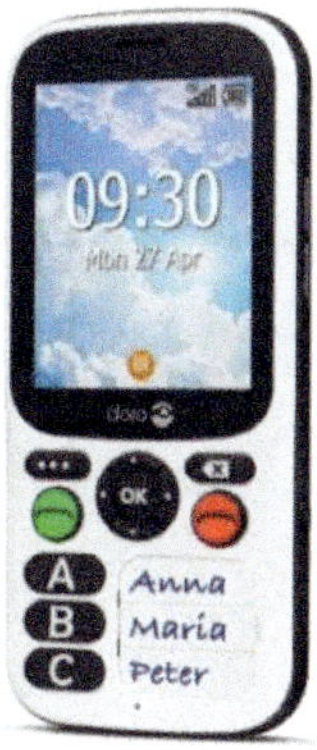

Doro 780x simple mobile phone features include SOS button that sends SMS and GPS message to friends and family who are set up to receive it. HAC (hearing aid compatible) and can be managed remotely

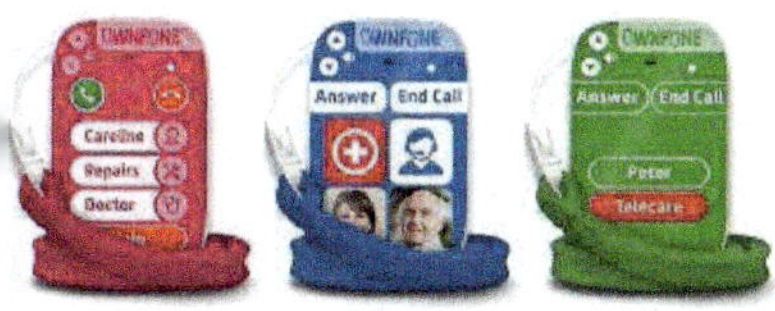

Ownfone This device allows the user to make calls to pre-programmed numbers, up to 12 and receive calls from anyone who has the number. You can design and customise the phone to tailor to an individual's needs.

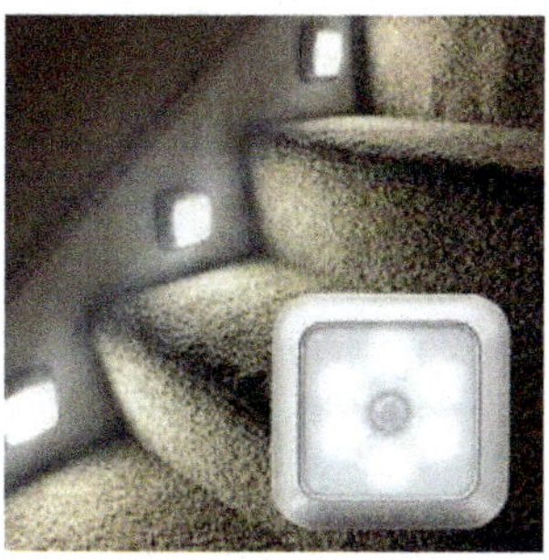

Battery powered light with movement sensor these devices can be used to light the way to the bathroom or simply to light up the stairway as a person approaches.

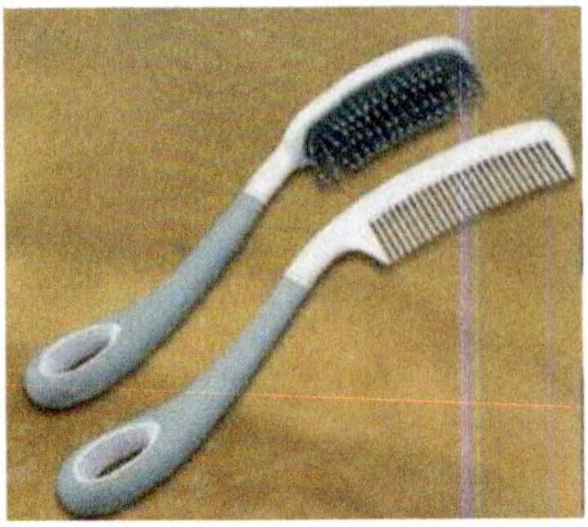

Long handled brush and comb – the long handled brush and comb can help a person to continue brush their hair when they start to struggle because they can no longer reach.

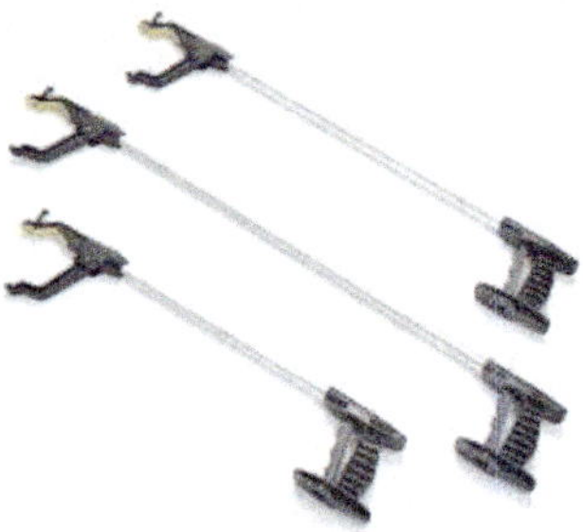

Helping hand/ grabber – the helping hand can help you to reach things without bending too much.

Case studies

George (aged 92 years old) receives help with food shopping and companionship for four hours per week. Having lost his wife to Alzheimer's, his main family contact is his stepdaughter Janet, who lives over 100 miles away. Janet wanted to be able to keep a regular eye on George's wellbeing, and not let their physical distance become a barrier. Janet logs into the sensor system that has been set up on a daily basis to check that George is alright. It begins with simply seeing whether he has been up in the night, and if he has made himself a cup of tea. Janet says: "It is great to have instant information available as living so far away from my stepdad can be difficult, but this technology means I can rest assured that he is safe and well". George says: "I barely notice that there are sensors in my house, and I know that it gives my stepdaughter comfort and reassurance."

Jean (aged 99 years old) received two care visits a day to support her as her needs increased. Her family are not local, so they had sensors installed to get a full view of Jean's activities around her home. The technology revealed that Jean was staying in bed longer than they realised, wasn't moving around in the house much, but was very active at night-time. This raised concerns about her susceptibility to having a fall. It seemed that Jean 'disappeared' for an hour every day at 4pm. Following investigation, Jean was recounting her school days during the blitz when her mother used to give her a glass of milk whilst Jean sat in the understairs cupboard. She was re-living this childhood experience. Using data from the sensors, Jean's family agreed to increase the number of care visits, particularly at 4pm to provide her with reassurance. With advice from her occupational therapist, Jean's bed was moved downstairs to avoid the possibility of her falling down the stairs at night. The family say: "Mum is very independent and has always been adamant that she will stay at home. Following the installation of sensors, we have been able to utilise the information it provides to fit care support around her increasing needs. The monitoring gives us immense reassurance that she is well, and Mum is happy that she can stay in her home where really she wants to be."

Questions and answers

Q1. My Mum who's in her sixties fell over last year on holiday in Spain and fractured her wrist. Should she be tested for osteoporosis?

A. Yes she should see her GP and discuss this. She may have slipped through the system as her fracture happened when she was abroad, though she would have been followed up by her local hospital when home. Sounds like she needs some blood tests and a bone density scan.

Q2. I'm really shocked. I've had three fractures in the last five years after I fell off my bike and had skiing accidents on two holidays. So I'm still staggering around using crutches waiting for my hip fracture to mend. That's bad enough, but I've just been told that I've got osteoporosis after having a bone scan, even though I'm only 55 years old and a man!

Now the hospital consultant says that I must take drugs for the rest of my life. So can I still cycle and ski, or should I just find new hobbies where I can sit down - and play chess perhaps?

A. The right exercises are what you need to be doing to build up your muscles to strengthen your bones and prevent falls, as well as taking regular bone strengthening drugs prescribed by your doctor like alendronic acid and top ups of calcium and vitamin D. There are special exercise programmes designed to strengthen your muscles and retrain your balance, to help you to maintain a steady gait. Try and do these everyday – a physiotherapist could teach you some reliable exercises. Exercise in measured ways, doing weight bearing exercises like running, skipping or dancing; resistance exercises such as press-ups or weightlifting might suit you too.

Chapter 8. So combat your back pain

Top tips

1. Think about your posture wherever you are, all day, everyday. If you're doing repetitive movements, or sitting or standing still for long periods, take activity breaks or stretch out frequently if you can.
2. If you're overweight then extra fat around your chest or middle can pull your spine out of position and trigger back pain. So guess what - if that's you, lose a few stone or you might have backache forever.
3. Look after your back at night. Go for a firm mattress so that your head, neck and spine are all supported. If the mattress is too hard, the natural curve of your spine will be overly straightened between your shoulders and hips. If your bed's too soft, you will sink into it and then your spine will curve unnaturally as an extended 'C' shape.

Most back problems can be avoided or minimised by adopting an appropriate posture whilst lifting or doing exercises. So, review your posture whilst working; if you must sit for a long-time during work hours, consider moving around periodically, and use appropriate workstations, chairs and accessories.

Some common things that you can do at home to prevent or manage back pain:

- A seat cushion to elevate a chair that you sit on. This will make it less stressful on your back to get up and sit down.
- Sometimes a firm surface on a chair seat is easier to get up from than a chair with a soft cushion.
- Within the kitchen, a high stool with back support can help to alleviate back pain.
- A modified and raised seat in the toilet with grab rails will reduce unnecessary stress on your lower back when you sit down or stand up.
- You can buy a back support to wear under your shirt or top in local shops or online.

- A grab bar in the bathroom will be supportive and helps to distribute your weight getting in and out of the bath.
- An appropriate length shoehorn allows you to put on shoes without bending and therefore reduces the strain on your back.

What is the pain?

Pain and muscle tightness or stiffness in the back between the lower ribs and the top of the legs is common and usually resolves itself over a period of time. Non-specific low back pain, muscle tension and stiffness originate from the bones or vertebrae of your spine, and/or the ligaments and muscles which are attached.

You might be pre-disposed to back pain because of being generally inactive, being overweight, having chronic health conditions, improper lifting or your work habits. Sometimes, more severe back pain might result from spinal problems such as a slipped disc, or a neurological problem such as sciatica.

Causes of back pain include:

- poor posture
- bad lifting techniques
- being overweight
- arthritis or wear and tear or spondylitis
- slipped or prolapsed disc
- osteoporosis.

Psychosocial factors including anxiety, depression and mental stress at work might make someone more prone to back pain if they're sitting around, hunched over. Many people developing low back pain are adults aged 20-55 years and are otherwise well.

Back pain is more likely in those people who do heavy physical work, frequent bending, twisting and lifting, suffer whole body vibration, or remain sitting in one position for a long time. The symptoms of backache or back pain depend on what the cause is, whether the pain arises from the spine and surrounding muscles, or whether a nerve is trapped at its root (sciatica or lumbago) so that pain radiates along the nerve.

Most backache is simply pain arising from the spine or muscles around the spine. 33 vertebrae make up your spine. They are joined together through your intervertebral discs - these cushion your spine and prevent it from jarring. The curved shape of your spine gives it strength and flexibility. Muscles and ligaments are attached to your spine too; these stabilise your spinal column.

The vertebrae each have a bony arch that link together to form the spinal canal – that runs down the length of your spine. Nerves pass from your brain to the rest of your body through this protective canal. Nerves to the legs are formed from the lumbar-sacral spine. Some of these join to make up the sciatic nerve, which supplies the leg and foot. Pain is triggered when the nerves are pressed on by your spine bones or attached muscles in your low back; and you may experience the pain shooting down the length of the nerve to your foot on one or both sides of your body.

Nerves that pass around your chest originate from your thoracic spine. Sometimes pain can be generated by pressure on the nerves as they leave the spine, and travel around towards your breastbone. Sometimes back pain in the thoracic spine in an older person can be due to osteoporosis, thinning of the bones.

A slipped disc is when the gel-like intervertebral disc is forced backwards or sideways to press on one or more nerve roots as they emerge from your spinal canal.

There are warning signs that someone has a serious back problem such as a prolapsed disc pressing on major nerves that operate their bowels and bladder. So these ‘red flags’ include anyone who loses control of their bladder or bowels or is numb around their buttocks and between their legs, or becomes very unsteady on their feet – and if they notice these symptoms and signs they should seek urgent medical help.

What you can do to prevent low back pain or minimise the pain

Take it easy for the first couple of days, move about gently, avoid bending forward, avoid strain and don't sit in a chair for any length of time.
Take painkillers like paracetamol or ibuprofen according to the manufacturer's instructions. A heat or ice pack applied to your lower back for around 30 minutes may help. Wrap ice packs in a towel.
Small amounts of exercise very frequently are best done within the limits of your back pain. If the pain persists, physical treatment from a physiotherapist, osteopath or chiropractor can help you to get moving.

Sensible lifting
Use machines and aids rather than lifting weights at work or home if you have a choice. Learn to lift properly and how to stand and sit with proper support. It may seem that 'lifting' is not an issue for you at home or work, but if you do not regularly make a physical effort, you are probably in a more vulnerable position if required to do so on an odd occasion, compared to someone else who handles heavy weights on a daily basis. Loads carried nearer the spine are easier to control, and create less strain on your spine – see some national recommendations in the box below:

Types of lifting	***Example recommended maximum weight***	
	Male	Female
-if lifting from below knee height, or above shoulder height if close to your body	10kg	7kg
-lifting at waist height close to your body	25kg	17kg

(if lifting involves twisting weight, then reduce maximum weights by 10 – 20%)
HSE Manual handling at work. A brief guide 2020.
https://books.hse.gov.uk

Regular exercise

Prevention is better than cure. Do regular exercise like walking, swimming or cycling but avoid sudden unaccustomed exercise which might start off a bout of back pain. Increase your fitness and strengthen your back muscles to guard against back pain recurring. If you do have an episode of back pain take it easy for the first couple of days, move about gently, avoid bending forward or straining your back and don't sit in a chair for too long. Small amounts of exercise very frequently are best. Specific exercises done within the limits of the pain can be helpful. Keep active and move around even if it hurts a bit.

Painkillers

Try a painkiller such as paracetamol or non-steroidal anti-inflammatory treatment such as ibuprofen that you can buy over the counter of a pharmacy (so long as you don't suffer from stomach problems), according to the manufacturer's instructions. Beware that non-steroidal tablets can give you indigestion – stop taking them if so as you don't want to end up with a stomach ulcer.

There are stronger painkillers such as those containing codeine if paracetamol gives you insufficient pain relief – maybe co-codamol (in varying strengths) or tramadol, (you can buy a weak codeine treatment over the counter from a pharmacy.) A stronger anti-inflammatory drug such as diclofenac might be prescribed by your doctor - so long as your stomach's up to it or you take prevention medication too.

An antidepressant drug might help if you've got chronic low back pain which has lasted for more than 12 weeks.

Heat or ice?

Try a heat or ice pack applied to the painful area of your back for around 10 (ice) or 20 (heat) minutes. Wrap the ice pack (maybe packet of frozen peas) in a tea towel. Or try a heat pad on the tender part of your low back.

TENS machine

Transcutaneous electrical nerve stimulation (TENS) could be worth trying as a way of relieving your low back pain (or other pain elsewhere).

They are sometimes used to try and help pregnant women with back pain when giving painkilling tablets or manipulating their back would be too dangerous, and their bulging pregnancy means that they can do few back exercises. TENS machines can be prescribed at some pain clinics, or you could buy one online.

Acupuncture
There is some research evidence that acupuncture relieves low back pain and improves function in the short term. The usual 'Western' approach is to insert a few fine needles (perhaps three or four) for around 20 minutes or so at traditional 'meridian' acupuncture points and also some trigger points – these are the sites of the most tender areas.

Chiropractic
Some people think that spinal manipulation does help to eliminate low back pain but does not necessarily get your back any more active than it would have been if you'd just got on with exercises and daily activities. Traction may help to relieve your pain by stretching the vertebrae and reducing pressure on the nerves, but there's no sure research evidence of this.

How hands on assistive devices might help back pain
Several simple assistive devices might help solve back pain issues. These include devices that help you with activities of daily living such as a long shoehorn, devices which will help you with stretching exercises or those to help you maintain good posture such as cushions for seats and supportive bed mattresses. There are also devices which provide orthotic support.

Another important element to consider is wearing appropriate footwear. Choose footwear that is comfortable (possibly with stretchable uppers) and supportive (possibly with appropriate cushioned insoles), possibly with elastic shoelaces that allow you to easily slide your foot in and out without having to strain to tie the laces. Appropriate footwear also helps you to maintain or increase your mobility and physical activity.

There are several off the shelf, back support braces and belts. These help in supporting and improving back posture which results in effective management of low back pain by unloading some of the weight applied to the back.

Ergonomics

Ergonomics is about improving the match between your job (at work or home) and your physical ability and workload capacity – combining comfort, health and productivity. Minimise the likelihood of triggering back pain by looking at your posture during your working day, with sensible lifting of any loads. Postural strains may be due to the working position that your job requires because of the furniture used.

Good posture is all about maintaining your spine and other joints in positions which create the least strain on your body. The natural curves of the spine should be preserved, so reducing disc compression and ligament strain, with other joints sufficiently well positioned so that any strain on ligaments and tendons is minimised.

Maintaining good posture is about co-ordinated action of various muscles working to maintain stability of your back or spine. The spine has three physiological curves:

- cervical curve – in the neck region which has a forward curvature.
- thoracic curve – in your upper and mid-back which has a backwards curvature.
- lumbar curve – in your lower back which has a forward curvature.

A good posture normally involves having your shoulder, hip, knee and ankle aligned in a straight line when seen from the side to reduce the amount of load placed on the joints, muscles and ligaments of your body and thus result in less strain.

There are commercial products called *posture correctors*. Some of these are effectively braces which maintain a specific position for your back. They support various parts of the back or the whole back. There are also some electronic devices which help train and maintain an upright posture. These tactile devices vibrate when you are in a bad posture so that you can adjust to maintain a good posture.

Another important part of the body which relates to your posture whilst sitting is your pelvis. The pelvis acts as the base for sitting and it should be stable. Any changes in the position of the pelvis affect your overall posture. There are several postural support devices available in the market to maintain a good posture and to support individuals to help improve their posture whilst sitting. These include appropriately designed seat base or cushions, properly angled backrests, armrests and footrests.

Postural strains can present problems when they occur many times in a day, or for long periods. It is easy for someone to reach into a stretched position once in a while, but if they do so for even quite a short period, strains can occur. So, while it may be no problem for you to bend down to knee height to collect a document emerging from a printer once, it could place an unreasonable strain on an administrator's back if they were to do this continuously for a quarter of an hour.

Postural strains may include the kind of working position required because of the furniture used, but they may also be related to the pace of your work, lack of rest periods, and work-related stress triggering musculoskeletal disorders.

Long periods spent looking at a computer screen and other similar equipment can lead to muscular and other physical problems, eye fatigue and maybe mental stress. These problems are minimised by installing a good quality ergonomic set up for a workstation, a person's working environment and tasks performed.

A lumbar support will help you to keep your spine in a good position. You might opt for a lumbar roll shaped support or other shaped cushion. Strap it to your chair at the right level. You can buy a lumbar support through your local pharmacy or from an online catalogue.

Avoid surgery

Pain clinics may try epidural injections and other invasive procedures – really just as a trial to help someone with severe chronic back pain. Advice has got to be – avoid surgery if possible. The trouble is that back pain is a symptom. It is difficult to be sure exactly what's causing it, even with all the clever technology that abounds today.

So you take a risk that surgery such as fusing some of your vertebrae together does not work- because your low back pain occurs for a different reason than the surgeon thought was the case, or that the operation does not correct the problem from where the pain is originating.

Simple ideas on improving ergonomics

Height and arrangement of shelves

- Does the filing system require staff to twist in order to see the names?
- Could rotating files or forward facing cabinets be used instead?
- Are shelves too high for the safe lifting of storage boxes? – either split up the contents into smaller parts which can be lifted safely, or use only shelves at a safe height.

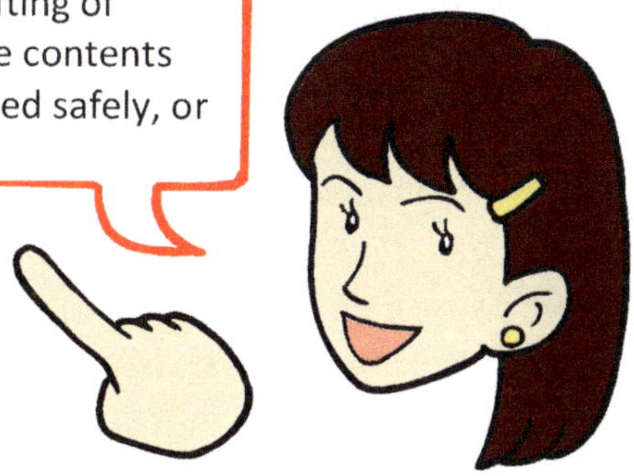

Avoid computer hump

Fix the height of your screen when working with any desktop or laptop computer so that it's parallel to your eyes and you're not looking up or down at it. Check that the height of your desk lets your shoulders relax and your elbows be positioned at right angles. Sit up straight close to your desk and square onto it. Adjust the height of your chair relative to your desk with your feet flat on the ground. It will really put your intervertebral discs under pressure if you have to elevate your arms to type on the keyboard. Sit up straight instead of slouching and putting strain on your back. Your wrists should be straight whilst you are tapping lightly on the keyboard. Sit square to the desk and computer screen. Keep your mouse near to your keyboard so that you don't have far to reach and can retain a good posture whilst you do so.

Using your computer

think of your

chair *footrest* *keyboard*

screen lighting *variation in tasks*

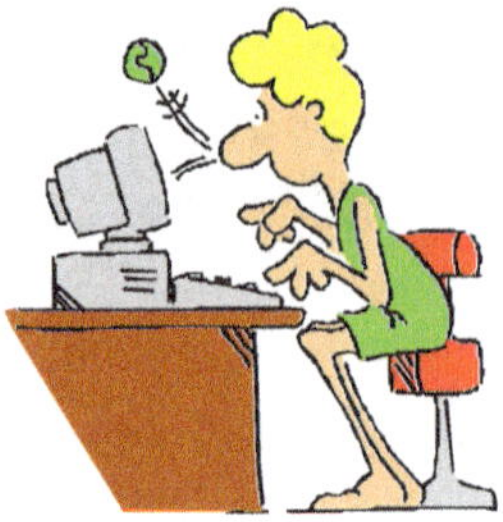

and consider if the guidance in the box below will help:

- adjustable height of seat and backrest on chair
- footrest available
- space around keyboard for wrist support, forearms are horizontal
- document holder positioned to minimise neck strain
- screen adjustable at optimum height
- (eyes level with top of screen, viewing display by looking at a slightly downwards angle)
- no glare, brightness adjusted for clear visibility
- other equipment used should be easily accessible without straining
- make sure there are no trailing cables
- work should allow frequent breaks or change in tasks to minimise strain.

Digital aids to help you combat your back pain

Not only can you search online for exercise, stretches or techniques to help you manage your back pain, but you can search online retailers for back and posture aids. There are many products available, from lumbar supports to back and waist straps.

The websites below give:

i) NHS advice about back pain

ii) a programme of back care exercises, which is essentially free, but for more detailed advice including live webinars, a monthly fee is required.

The video provides a good description of current thinking about the knowledge and treatment of back pain, together with patients' views.

Websites	Videos
NHS Back Pain	**Advice and patient experience about back pain**

'Have a healthy back' is a series of mobilisation exercises from an NHS physiotherapist.

Website with free or paid subscription:

www.backinshapeprogram.com

Have a Healthy Back

Then there are two videos about McKenzie back exercises, which have been used widely and successfully in many countries, including the UK. The first video is by two physios from the USA, who describe the principles of the McKenzie methods, then the McKenzie exercises to be done at home are shown in a less flamboyant way by a different physio. The app is one of many which give exercises to help strengthen, mobilise, and maintain the back, but professional advice should be sought before using these exercises while in a lot of pain.

McKenzie Back Exercise principles

McKenzie Exercises at home

App

Back pain exercises at home

Apple

Play Store

Smart Speaker

- Set a timer for your stretches or exercises
- Use workout or training skills to guide you through exercises
- Set yourself a reminder to sit-up straight in your chair at work or home.

Search term keywords and phrases:

- back pain relief
- morning stretching routines
- chair exercises
- yoga class
- posture aid

Case studies

Dan had been a keen gardener all his adult life but aged 80 years old felt that he couldn't carry on anymore as he got such back ache bending down and tending to his plants.
But everything improved when he met a friend out for a walk with their daughter, Kerry, a physiotherapist. She advised him that when gardening he must watch his back. She told him "Bend your knees and not your back when you're digging and weeding. Kneel down when you're planting out, so you can keep your back straight instead of bending over." He did this and also set up raised beds for growing his plants. So he's careful to follow Kerry's advice & has managed to comfortably keep going with his gardening.

Deidre had to travel long distances at work as part of her sales work to various factories and company meetings and found that the regular car journeys of three or so hours were crippling her, with the back pain it was generating. She was thinking of looking for another job; but then the COVID pandemic struck and her sales meetings were re-booked as virtual catch ups via Zoom meetings. She found that joining the sales meetings by video conferencing or telephone group discussions worked just as well as those she used to attend in person. She uses a lumbar support strapped to her chair to help to keep her spine in a good position when she's sitting at her desk on her laptop; and gets up and strolls round her house and garden between virtual meetings. So her back pain has settled down, and she still has the same sales job and very infrequent back pain now.

Questions and answers

Q1. I'm full of aches and pains especially at the end of my working week in a supermarket when stacking shelves. How can I minimise my aches and back pains?

A. Learn to lift properly and try not to stand still for too long. Sit with proper support. Good posture helps to maintain your spine and other joints in positions which create least strain. By preserving the natural curves of your spine you'll reduce compression of your intervertebral discs or strain on your ligaments. Prevention is better than cure so do regular exercise like walking, swimming, cycling but avoid sudden unaccustomed exercise which might trigger muscle or joint pain.

Q2. I get awful backache at the office, sitting for hours on end working on the computer or answering customers' queries by phone. What can I do?

A. Get a firm, high backed chair to sit upright in. Sit up properly on the chair and try a small cushion to support your lower lumbar spine. If that chair supports your head and neck too that's even better. If your job involves standing for long periods, try to adjust the height of your working surface to a comfortable level. Your employer should undertake an 'ergonomics' assessment of what chair and desk set up will suit you and make back problems less likely. Then kit you out with the right chair and desk – ask them for help.

Chapter 9. Building your muscle and/or joints & overcoming pain

Top tips

1. Muscle and joint pains from sports injuries are common but it may not be until the day after the sports activity that you realise you've strained your muscle or inflamed your joints - so people can be confused as to what the actual cause was.
2. Although joint pain gets increasingly more common as people get older it is not an inevitable consequence of ageing. Although it may be something you have to *live with*, you should not have to *suffer from* it.
3. Osteoarthritis is sometimes described as 'wear and tear' of your joints. But it's more like 'wear and repair' as the joints in your body are constantly adapting to the various stresses on them – from an injury or overuse or maybe the weight they need to support if you're too heavy and could do with dropping to a healthy weight.

The symptoms of aching or pain depend on what the cause is, whether the pain arises from an overstrained muscle or an inflamed joint or whether a nerve is trapped at its root, so that pain radiates down the nerve to your arm or leg or shoulder and so on.

Non-specific muscular pain, tension and stiffness originates from your bones and/or the ligaments and muscles which are attached. Or pain may arise from a nerve as it comes out of the spine or another joint and is trapped at its root so that pain shoots along the nerve. Joint swelling is a consequence of the inflammation.

Muscle and joint pain is more likely in those people who do heavy physical work, frequent bending down, twisting and lifting, or remain in one position for a long time. The inflammation leading to joint pain is often triggered by repetitive movements or trauma from work or hobbies.

A common cause of recurrent or longer-term (e.g. over 3 months) joint pain as you get older is osteoarthritis. Typical symptoms of osteoarthritis are:

- joint swelling
- pain and/or stiffness
- pain that is worse on moving or after a period of inactivity.

Osteoarthritis most commonly affects your knees, hips, spinal joints and hands. When severely affected, the joint space is narrowed and osteophytes form (little bony spikes) with some bone changes so that generates pain as the main bones rub together.

People usually start to suffer from osteoarthritis between the ages of 45 and 55 years and most people over 75 years old, will have some degree of osteoarthritis in their various joints. There is a lot you can do to help yourself and your joints can improve over time and become unaffected or symptom free. Joints that are commonly affected by osteoarthritis are the finger joints, base of the thumb, knees and hips. However it can occur anywhere and is more likely to occur in joints that have been previously injured.

Usually osteoarthritis is diagnosed by how someone describes the pain or swelling of their joint(s) and how swollen the joint looks and feels, rather than the extent of structural changes seen on an Xray of the joint(s). Sometimes diagnosing osteoarthritis is confused by other musculoskeletal disorders that a person might have too - like gout or fibromyalgia.

There are a variety of treatments for osteoarthritis. The simplest is for a person to self care. So that would be weight reduction if they're overweight, muscle strengthening exercises, walking aids, taping the patellar joint of their knee to provide more support, and adding insoles to their footwear. Just wearing supporting cushioned trainers may make an enormous difference to daily walking if you have osteoarthritis in your feet.

Someone who needs pain relief for their osteoarthritis should try paracetamol or rub in anti-inflammatory cream that they've bought over

Digital aids to help you to build your muscles and joints

Website	Video	App
How to improve your strength and flexibility	**NHS Fitness studio**	**7-minute workout** Apple Playstore

Smart Speaker

Search term keywords and phrases:

- muscle pain relief
- morning stretching routines
- chair exercises
- yoga class

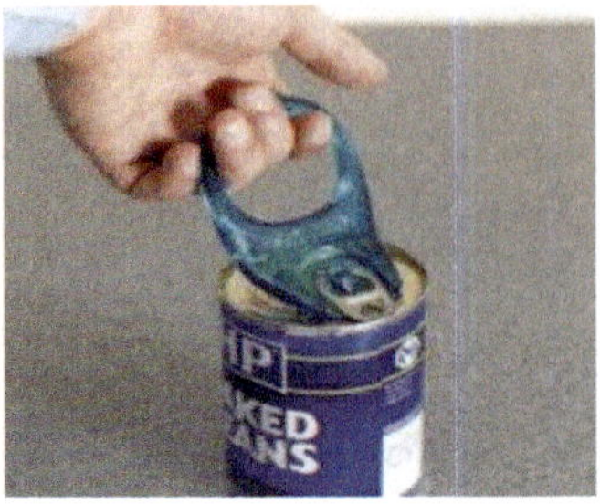

Can Pull - Ring pull can opener. Hook is slipped under ring and angled forwards to raise the ring and then angled backwards to pull on the ring to open.

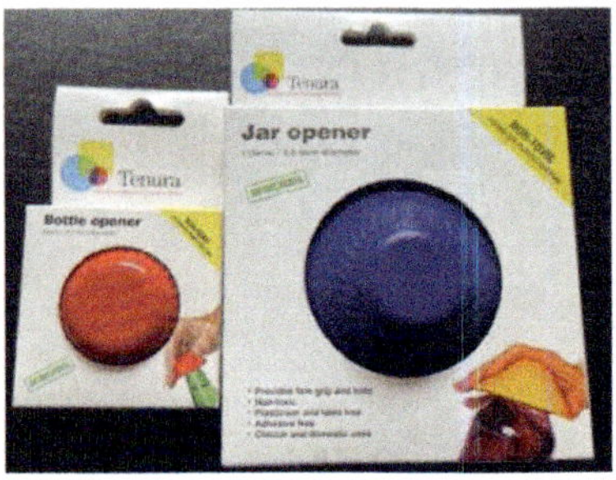

Twister Jar Opener - These dome shaped openers grip jar and bottle lids. They are made from a flexible slip-resistant material which, when placed over the lid of a jar or bottle, may enhance the users grip on the lid. These products can be light weight compared to openers with handles or adjustable gripping surfaces. https://www.youtube.com/watch?v=e6WJ0o_Se_E

Case studies

Dave had an awful whiplash injury when a car suddenly shunted forcibly into the back of his car whilst he was stationery in a traffic queue. It didn't hurt too much on the day but the next morning he went to A&E as he was in agony – he had looked up medical advice online but still felt he wanted an expert clinical view in person. After examining him thoroughly the A&E consultant, Mr Din explained that his neck pain was due to the overstretching or ripping of his neck muscles and associated ligaments after the sudden neck jerk movement backwards when the other car bashed into his car. Mr Din said it was common in that circumstance for someone's neck to feel reasonably comfortable when the trauma happens - and then the pain can really hit home the next day – with pain radiating from their neck over their head, across their shoulders and down their arm, often one sided depending on the nature of the trauma and how it happened. Dave felt reassured and tried to tolerate the neck pain for the next few days with heat and ice pads, a neck-support pillow, paracetamol & his wife massaging the area. Two weeks later he was completely better and not needing pain relief anymore.

Mary has had pain in the soles of her feet when she walks half a mile or so for as long as she can remember – since she was 50 years old anyway. She went to see a podiatrist for the first time when she was 60 years old. He examined Mary and pushed her to look after herself better – and self care. So that included losing weight (Mary needed to lose two stones to fit into the 'ideal' weight category so that her body mass index was less than 25), muscle strengthening exercises for her feet and legs in general (Mary started swimming three times a week), and adding insoles to her footwear (he recommended specific gel insoles which Mary bought and fitted in her daily walking shoes). Mary found that just wearing supporting cushioned trainers made an enormous difference to the comfort of her daily walking – and now the pain in the soles of her feet is much diminished.

Questions and answers

Q1. I have such aches and pains in my knees which my doctor says are due to osteoarthritis. I can't take ibuprofen tablets anymore as they give me heartburn and paracetamol is not strong enough. What else can I do to help and enable me to keep on walking with my dog everyday?

A. Have you tried ibuprofen gel or another anti-inflammatory such as voltarol emugel that you can buy in a shop or pharmacy. They could be the answer for you. It's thought that only about 6% of the gel is absorbed in the bloodstream compared to swallowing it as a tablet, so it's much less likely that the gel you apply triggers heartburn or even worse, stomach bleeding. You could also try cold compresses or ice packs held around your knees for say five minutes, two or three times a day.

Q2. My father is in his 80s and a keen gardener. But he lives on a steep hill and he's finding it difficult to manage the steps and kneel down to weed because bending his knees is really painful. What treatment do you suggest?

A. You're best getting an occupational therapist's advice on what tools he could use to grip better and stand more steadily. It'll be better to sit on a low portable chair to do the weeding rather than kneel down. Setting up rails to help him up and down the steps is really important so he doesn't fall and stays active.

Q3. I've had pain from the muscles in my arms and legs for years. My GP has increased my painkillers and I've tried paracetamol, ibuprofen and strong codeine tablets - but none of them work well and I've had to give up my job in a shop and retire early. I've just been given amitriptyline to try but reading the leaflet, I see that it's to treat depression. Does my doctor think that I'm just depressed and not believe me when I describe the terrible pain I get everyday?

A. Amitriptyline is used for pain relief at lower doses than those used for depression. So at this dose, it is used to treat neurological, longstanding pain. Anticonvulsant drugs are sometimes used for pain relief too. They are prescribed in similar doses to relieve pain as for controlling fits. It's worth giving it a try!

Chapter 10. Get tech help if visually impaired

Top tips

1. Virtually all technology devices available today have an array of built-in accessibility options, which help people who may be hard of hearing or visually impaired. Check the vision, hearing, physical and motor options such as voice control, magnifier, display and text size, sound recognition, face ID – and make sure that your device is set up correctly to suit your needs.
2. Many smartphones now have a digital assistant built in and can be accessed by using your voice.
3. You can probably manage simple eye problems such as not being able to read as small print as you used to, or when your eyelashes are stuck together with messy discharge, or just seem sore and dry or even itchy, yourself without needing a doctor's or optician's help. But for more serious eye problems like cataracts, glaucoma, damage to the retina at the back of the eye, a stroke or migraine, a doctor's or optometrist's diagnosis & treatment will be critical.

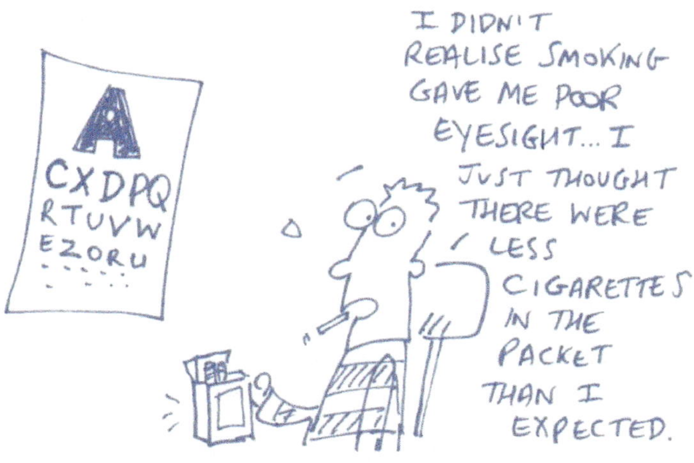
A
CXDPQ
RTUVW
EZORU
I DIDN'T REALISE SMOKING GAVE ME POOR EYESIGHT... I JUST THOUGHT THERE WERE LESS CIGARETTES IN THE PACKET THAN I EXPECTED.

Eye problems to look out for

Eye problems are commonplace – such as not being able to read as small print as you used to, or when your eyelashes are stuck together with messy discharge, or they just seem sore and dry or even itchy. These are all conditions that you can probably manage yourself without needing a doctor's or optician's help. There are other more serious eye problems like cataracts, glaucoma, damage to the retina at the back of the eye, a stroke or migraine where medical diagnosis and treatment will be critical.

The place to go when you notice you're having progressively more difficulty reading is your local optician (sometimes called optometrist). They can examine your eyes in-depth and gauge your vision and the pressure in both of your eyes and see if you need further investigations. They can recommend the strength and type of glasses or contact lenses you need and provide these. Or you can buy a cheaper version of those glasses at a retail store.

If you notice that your eyelashes are a bit crusty or you have some mucky discharge in the corner of an eye you are likely to have a bit of an infection. If you wash your closed eyelids with salty water a few times for two days, the infection's likely to clear up. If it persists you can buy an antibiotic cream to put into your eye(s) several times a day over the counter from your local pharmacy. But if it's still mucky a week later go to see your GP.

When people get dry eyes they seem uncomfortable and sore. It's more likely to happen as people grow older or as a result of being in a windy environment such as from air conditioning. It can be due to a medical condition such as Sjogren's syndrome which is an auto-immune disorder, or Parkinson's disease. Dry eyes can be a side effect of some types of medication too – look at the information leaflet that comes with your prescribed or shop bought medication. First off you can buy hypromellose 0.3% eye drops or Viscotears liquid gel over the counter of a pharmacy and avoid any allergens, then see if that relieves your sore eyes.

You might have dry eyes too from an allergy such as pollen in the hayfever season or other things that you're allergic to, such as perfumes or animal hair. Try to avoid those allergens as far as you can - like not going for a country walk when the pollen count is high. You can buy eye drops with an antihistamine in such as azelastine to see if its regular application relieves your itch and soreness.

Digital aids to help you to help with visual impairment

Accessibility features

To find out more about accessibility options and how to turn them on you can visit the phone manufacturers' websites for tutorials and guides. The two most popular ones, Apple and Android, are linked below.

Apple	Android
https://www.apple.com/uk/accessibility	https://support.google.com/accessibility/android

Some new technology is being developed to help with visual impairment when out shopping:

Google **Lookout** app uses artificial intelligence to identify objects through image recognition – but the results are reported to be not fully perfect.

Supersense reads out aloud any text you hover the phone's camera over over, and can also read barcodes on food packages.

Be My Eyes allows users to call for assistance from volunteers who help to identify objects via video call.

Braille is applied to the packaging of many products, particularly medicines, deodorants and cleaning liquids.

Navilens Digital Codes are a new development, where manufacturers print coloured sqared codes onto packaging, and using an app on a smartphone, together with the phone's camera, arrange that information can be provided by audio to the partially sighted person. At present, these are mainly available on breakfast cereals, but more manufacturers are likely to follow this lead.The advantage is that the codes can be read from a distance of up to three metres, and their use could be widespread - to transport information, on any packaging of goods for sale, or instructions – the list is limitless.

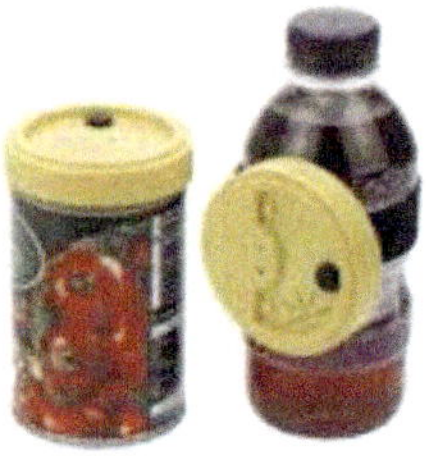

Talking tins – These help people with a visual impairment to identify the contents of their tinned food. Record a message of up to 10 seconds of what is in the tin, then play it back at the touch of a button.

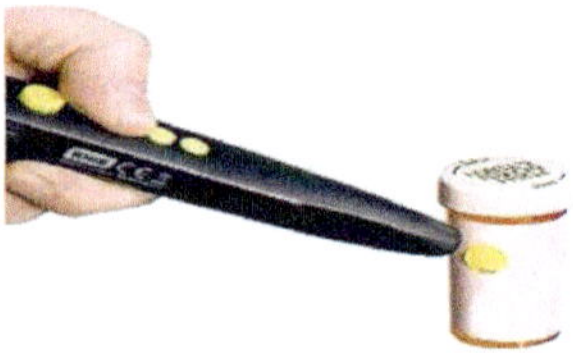

Pen friend voice labeller – Once set up the pen friend can be used to identify different products by scanning the sticky labels.

Dementia gradually affects an individual's ability to:

- remember things for more than a few seconds
- understand situations
- cope with everyday tasks
- express feelings
- think clearly in order to solve problems
- cope with an over-stimulating environment
- behave in the 'normal ways' they have learned throughout their lives
- make decisions
- understand the sequence of complex tasks, eventually being unable to perform simple tasks without help.

About five per cent of people in the UK over 65 years and 20% of those over 80 years have some sort of dementia.

Essentially dementia is characterised by a triad of changes which are:
1. Loss of memory
2. Loss of another aspect of cognition
3. Impairment of everyday life.

There are many types of dementia but the two most common types in older people are Alzheimer's disease and multi-infarct dementia (also known as vascular dementia). Both of these types of dementia are irreversible and cannot be cured, although their deterioration may be slowed down with prescribed drugs if given at an early enough stage.

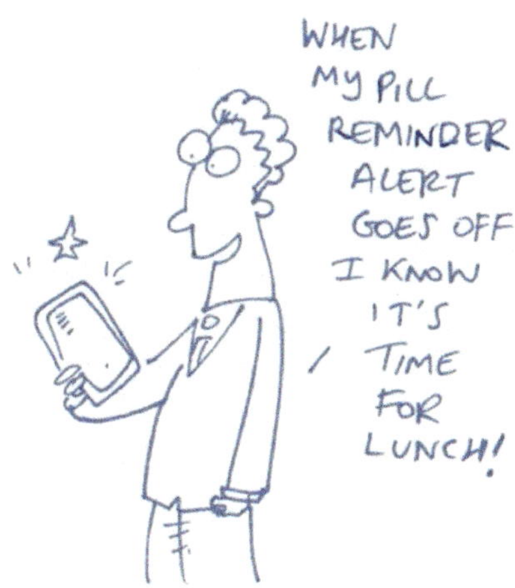
WHEN MY PILL REMINDER ALERT GOES OFF I KNOW IT'S TIME FOR LUNCH!

Alzheimer's disease is the fourth most common cause of death in the Western world, after heart disease, cancer and strokes. Over half of all dementia patients in the UK have this type. The main features are: prominent and progressive memory impairment, conversational problems such as difficulties finding the right words, disorientation in place particularly in unfamiliar surroundings and global cognitive impairment.

Vascular dementia is the second most common type of dementia. The person with it suffers damage to small areas of the brain, sometimes following a stroke or from a series of small strokes. This damage can lead to vascular dementia. Alzheimer's disease and multi-infarct dementia can occur together. Features suggesting vascular dementia include a recent history of a cerebrovascular accident, transient ischaemic attack or myocardial infarction, the presence of vascular risk factors or focal neurological signs (may indicate other causative conditions too). Vascular dementia develops in a step like way as little vascular events happen, the damage depending on which area of the brain is affected. The risk factors for vascular dementia are other health conditions that include: hypertension, diabetes, smoking, previous cerebrovascular accident or transient ischaemic attack and atrial fibrillation. About 80% of the people who have had Parkinson's disease for ten years or more have cognitive impairment.

Dementia is classified according to the varying degrees of minimal, mild, moderate and severe dementia that merge into each other.

Minimal dementia
A person with 'minimal' dementia has some difficulty in recalling recent events and may be prone to mislaying or losing things. A person with minimal dementia is usually still able to be independent and care is probably not needed.

Mild dementia
A person with 'mild' dementia has most of the following signs and symptoms: difficulty in recalling recent information; limited or patchy disorientation in time and place; impaired problem solving, reasoning and the ability to manage everyday activities.

In the later stages of mild dementia some degree of care will usually be required.

Moderate dementia
A person with 'moderate' dementia has most of the following signs and symptoms: severely impaired reasoning, problem solving and recall of recent events; disorientated in time and place; speech slightly unclear, but not to a marked degree; not able to manage housework, shopping and finances independently; help with dressing and other self-care; be occasionally incontinent. Daily care is usually required for those with moderate dementia.

Severe dementia
A person with 'severe' dementia is totally disorientated, incapable of recall, reasoning and self-care, unable to communicate in normal speech, may fail to recognise close relatives, is almost invariably incontinent, apathetic and inert. The person with severe dementia may become immobile, and will be totally incapable of being independent. Continual care and supervision are usually required.

The need for care depends on how long an individual can remain living alone or being independent. The needs of an individual tend to vary from time to time, as there may be episodes of severely disturbed behaviour. So health and social care services need to be flexible.

People with dementia live for about seven or eight years on average after the problem has been first diagnosed, although there are wide individual variations. They and their families have to deal with the effects of dementia itself - not only the deterioration in memory, reasoning and ability but also the changes in relationships and interactions as other people begin to treat them differently. The most difficult problems for carers to cope with are personality changes in their dementing dependants, lack of everyday conversation, criticism, excessive demands and difficult behaviour such as aggression, disturbance at night, incontinence and wandering off.

If you're still wondering if you or someone you know might have the beginnings of dementia after reading this chapter, match your symptoms to the 'healthy' or 'mild dementia' column in the Table below. If you think you or they may have mild dementia, go and consult your GP.

Table 11.1. Comparison of memory and cognition in healthy people with those with mild dementia

	Healthy	**Mild dementia**
Memory	Occasional lapses	Impaired memory for recent events
Orientation	Fully orientated in time, space and person	Variable disorientation in time and place
Judgement and problem solving	Solves everyday problems	Some difficulty with complex problems
Outside home	Independent functioning	Engaged in some activities but not independently
At home	Activities and interests maintained	More difficult tasks and hobbies abandoned
Personal care	Fully capable	Needs some prompting to undertake everyday living activities

What can be done to prevent dementia happening or getting worse?

Early diagnosis will allow the person to reduce their risk factors such as stopping smoking, gaining better control over their raised blood pressure, diabetes or heart disease. Aspirin may help to prevent further vascular events in patients with a previous history of transient ischaemic attack or stroke if judged to be safe to be taken by their responsible clinician (because aspirin can cause bleeding).

Specific prescribed drugs can delay a person's cognitive decline; others help to modify any behavioural and psychiatric disturbances and symptoms such as depression, delusions, hallucinations and wandering off.

Specialist assessment and follow up is required to agree and provide the range of treatment, support and care as the dementia runs its course with individually tailored care plans that help carers and health professionals address a person's deteriorating memory functioning and behaviour. The chosen treatment plan should be developed and reviewed at appropriate intervals.

People with dementia may need medication for other health problems too that are entirely separate from, or associated with, their dementia, or worsening of their deterioration. People with dementia who also have a depressive disorder should be offered antidepressants. If a person with dementia seems to be in pain, then painkillers may reverse their unexplained changes in behaviour and/ or signs of distress.
Better medical control of an unduly raised blood pressure or high blood sugar levels from diabetes or high cholesterol levels in their blood, should hopefully slow down someone's deterioration from dementia.

There are a range of non-drug treatments that can help to minimise behavioural problems and assist in the overall care of people with dementia:

- for people with dementia who have agitation: aromatherapy, multisensorial stimulation, massage, animal assisted therapy, and therapeutic use of music and dance may help.
- behavioural interventions: the exact options depend on what type of behavioural problems need to be addressed.
- occupational activities to stimulate them.
- environmental modifications making the person's home safer; reminding them to take their medication etc.
- reminiscence helping their memory recall. Surround someone with familiar objects that can be used to stimulate their memory. Other materials, such as family scrapbooks, flash cards, favourite games, a world globe, large-piece jigsaw puzzles, and illustrated books might also help.
- regular exercise to help the person stay fit and minimise their vascular risks.

People with memory impairment or dementia should be encouraged to perform activities of daily living as far as possible for themselves - such as getting dressed, eating, taking care of personal hygiene and be complimented on their attempts and achievements.

Digital aids to help you with a diminishing memory

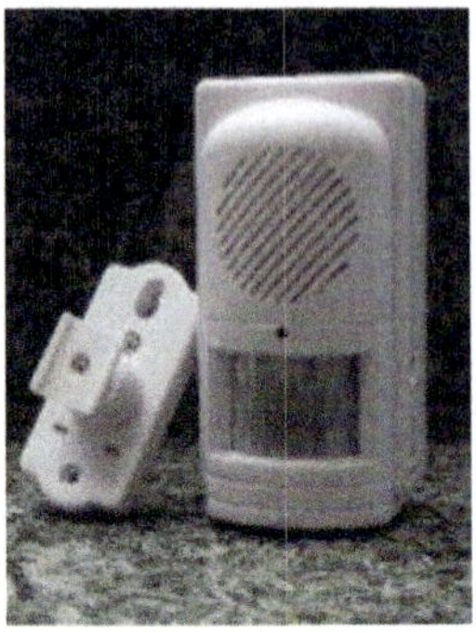

Memo-minder - You might find the Memo-minder helpful if you live on your own and you're worried that your memory problems could put you in an unsafe position, such as leaving your house without your keys and accidently locking yourself out. Activated by a passive motion detector the Memo-minder is usually mounted by the front door and when activated will play a message which could be pre-recorded by a friend or family member so it's a familiar voice you will hear.
https://www.youtube.com/watch?v=X4GkxV2Zv3A

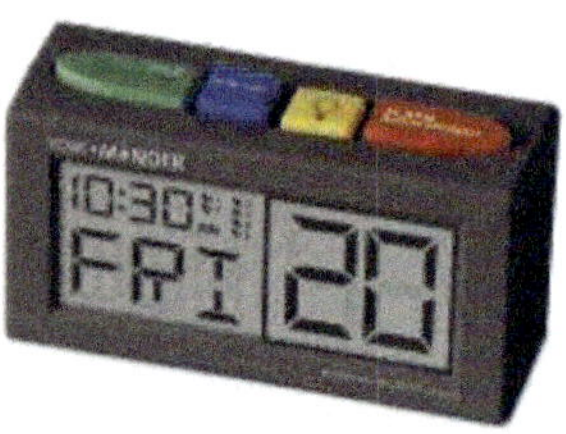

Talking reminder clock – a talking clock with announcements of time, day and date, six recordable daily prompts of ten seconds each which repeat for 60 seconds or until stopped. It can be battery or mains powered.

https://www.youtube.com/watch?v=TDjwfGSp2ak

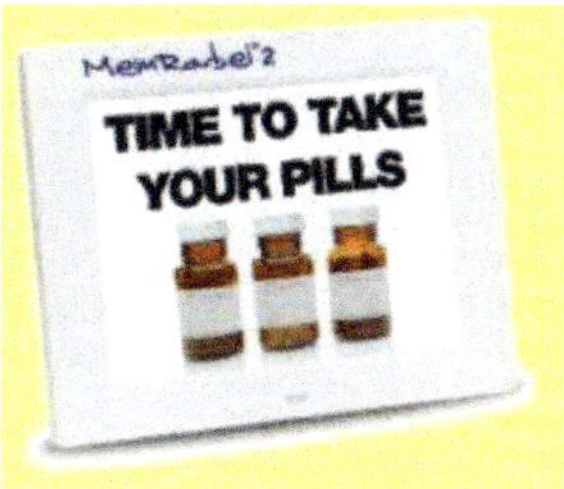

Memrabel 2 - Electric photo frame that can be programmed to provide alarm reminders with graphics, video or audio – relevant to taking medication, appointments with doctor or dentist, meeting up with friends or family.
https://www.youtube.com/watch?v=7bePn3KlUUQ

Take a look at these tech aids:

Website	Video	App	
Alzheimer's Society	**Power Foods for the Brain, Neal Barnard | TEDxBismarck**	**Clear dementia care** Apple	Play store

Smart speaker

Smart speakers can be really useful for someone with cognitive impairment. Useful features include:

- reminders (these can be for anything, and repeated daily, weekly or monthly etc.)
- lists that can be made and recalled at any time.
- playing music
- video or voice calling
- smart speakers with a screen that can be used as a digital photo frame, which can be really useful for memory recall.

Video streaming: Videos and music are great ways to reignite memories and YouTube is a great source for both.

Apps

There are thousands of apps to help stimulate the mind. From simple puzzle games to more complex problem solving and brain training, there will always be something to suit a person's needs.

Other online resources

https://www.meetadam.co.uk/ Meet Adam is an online website for those living with, or caring for, someone with dementia. The site provides valuable information around all sorts of technology available to keep someone safe and independent in their own home.

Case studies

When **Anna** received her Echo Show device for her birthday from her daughter Cath, her family realised how much *Alexa* could aid Anna with her severe memory loss. Often forgetting various common things was causing Anna extreme stress and anxiety in her everyday living. This was alleviated through *Alexa*'s ability to provide her with reminders, timers and alarms, and earn Anna's trust that she could rely upon the technology offered. A further unexpected outcome was that Anna's daughter Cath was deaf, and as she lived 50 miles away from her mother they weren't able to communicate very often. The Echo Show now allows them both to engage in video-calls, enabling Cath to lip read what Anna says and participate in conversation. This outcome has been a fantastic way to reduce social isolation for both Anna and Cath. Furthermore, Cath purchased her own *Alexa* device to have in her home, enabling quicker and simpler access to vital communication between mother and daughter.

John wanted to agree 'Advanced care planning' whilst he still had the mental capacity to make a decision. (This is a process of discussion between a patient and health or social care professional and sometimes their family carers.) He ended up with:

1. An advanced statement expressing his preference for his future care
2. A living will: making an informed decision to refuse certain treatments in specific conditions, if he suffered a further loss of mental capacity in the future.
3. A lasting power of attorney: he named his oldest son Brian to act on his behalf if he lost capacity in future in elation to his health and/ or financial matters.

Although John realised that he only had mild dementia, he felt much more reassured knowing that these documents were all agreed and in place with his oldest son prepared to take responsibility for helping him, if and when his dementia grew worse.

Questions and answers

Q1. I'm really worried about my husband, Chris, who's aged 81 years old. He's been behaving strangely over the last year or two. Since he backed our car into a lamp-post, I've tried to persuade him to stop driving but then he loses his temper and shouts at me. Last week, a light bulb went in the hall and he didn't know how to change it even though he's done so for decades. When I told him to leave it, he became really aggressive and threw the screwdriver at me. Has he got dementia? What can we do?

A. In the early stages of dementia, people may deny that anything is wrong. In the later stages, people are usually unaware that they have any disability. Make an appointment with your GP (a double appointment if that's possible as you'll need plenty of time) and go along with Chris. You can both then capture what's been happening. Your GP will do some screening and blood tests and likely refer Chris to a specialist to investigate possible causes further and start him on the right treatment.

Q2. My mother, Freda who's aged 72 years old, went bonkers last month. I took her to the doctor's. It turned out she had a urine infection and she's a lot better now. We're worried she's developing dementia though – could she be?

A. It is common for a urine infection to trigger confusion in an older person, which doesn't happen usually in younger people. So if Freda's memory and behaviour are back to normal and there's a good reason she was confused because of her urine infection, then that doesn't seem like she has dementia – though will be good if she has a review at her doctor's to check her memory and cognition.

Chapter 12. So combat your sleep problems

Top tips

1. Adopt a healthy lifestyle and improve your sleep – no smoking, regular exercise, limited alcohol, avoid caffeine containing drinks, not eating too much or too late but not going to bed hungry.
2. Cognitive behavioural therapy can help you to sleep better – by avoiding unhelpful ways of thinking that can make you more anxious and interfere with your sleep; it's available online.
3. Recent research looking at hundreds of thousands of adults in the USA has shown that sleeping for around seven hours a day on average gives you health benefits; people who have far too much or too little sleep as their norm are more likely to die of heart disease, cancer and other ill-health.

What are the issues?

A good restful sleep is vital to your physical and emotional wellbeing. If your sleep's disturbed, you'll feel irritable and down next day, and find it difficult to concentrate at work.

Insomnia is the term that describes poor quality sleep, with difficulty getting off to sleep or staying asleep, waking too early in the morning, or not feeling refreshed when you waken up. It's a common problem. Nearly half of all adults suffer from it, some more than others. Disturbed sleep over a prolonged period of time on at least three nights a week reduces your quality of life.

How it happens

Don't expect to have the same instantaneous, deep sleep you had as a youngster as you get older. It's normal for your sleep to be lighter and shorter and more fragmented as you grow older. What matters really is how fatigued you are during the daytime due to your disturbed sleep, or how much your concentration is impaired or your mood altered.

Sometimes there are other health problems or conditions that disturb your sleep - such as depression, pain that keeps you awake or dementia - when people wander around through the night.

Severe snoring can result in a disturbed sleep pattern. Obstructive sleep apnoea is an extreme version; due to recurrent and frequent complete obstruction of the airway passing through the pharynx (back of mouth/throat). You can actually stop breathing 500-600 times in one night. If you think you might have this condition, you'll need to consult a doctor about this.

What you can do yourself to minimise sleep problems

- It's got to be regular exercise. Getting physically tired should help you to sleep - you should be aiming for at least 30 minutes of moderate exercise on at least five days of the week anyway for good health. It might be worth trying a walk before dinner – in a safe area of town; or perhaps a 20 - 30 minutes stint on your exercise bike at home.
- Avoid alcohol – drinking excessively is out.
- Avoid heavy meals in the evening - try having a main meal at lunchtime and a lighter meal in the early evening.
- Avoid caffeine containing drinks - especially from the early evening onwards – it gets your heart racing and triggers you into feeling really alert.
- Don't let yourself drop off with daytime naps - they can mess up your sleep pattern. Stay awake - if you're feeling drowsy jump up and do something active.
- Consider if any prescribed drugs or medicines you've bought over the counter might be disturbing your sleep and see if you can stop taking them or switch to an alternative drug. A drug like simvastatin for instance, taken to reduce a high cholesterol blood level, can cause sleep problems as a side effect.
- Don't get fixated about having a solid 'eight' hours sleep. Everyone's needs are different, and it's not an ideal world where you have the time or opportunity to sleep undisturbed for such a protected time. Get into the mindset that the amount of sleep you need is enough to enable you to feel refreshed and able to function effectively the following day. That could be as little as 5 or 6 hours for some people; 8 or 9 hours for others. Cut down on disturbances whilst you're asleep by creating a calm bedroom environment. Turn off your phone, put your pet to sleep where you don't hear its incidental noises, fix up blackout curtains if

sunlight disturbs you in the early morning, or wear ear plugs if you've a noisy partner snoring next to you. Get a comfortable bed and firm pillow, and ensure that you're not too hot from your bedding. If your bed is uncomfortable buy a firmer mattress, or put a board under your mattress.

- Establish a regular sleep habit and a regular routine with certain rituals (e.g. a warm bath) whilst getting ready to go to bed, going to bed at a regular time, and not staying in bed if you're unable to drop off to sleep after a reasonable time - say 45 minutes. Get up and do something for a short time rather than lie there tossing and turning and getting frustrated before trying again to drop off asleep.
- Lose weight if you're obese. The fat round your neck can press on your airway and make snoring worse - and that in turn can disturb your sleep.
- Don't work too late at night. This will just get your brain overactive and it will take an hour or more to wind down.
- Sex may help you to sleep - a nice ending to the day, with an automatic feeling of relaxation after intercourse is over, basking in your partner's love.
- If you've a noisy partner you could wear ear plugs or get them to try snoring aids.

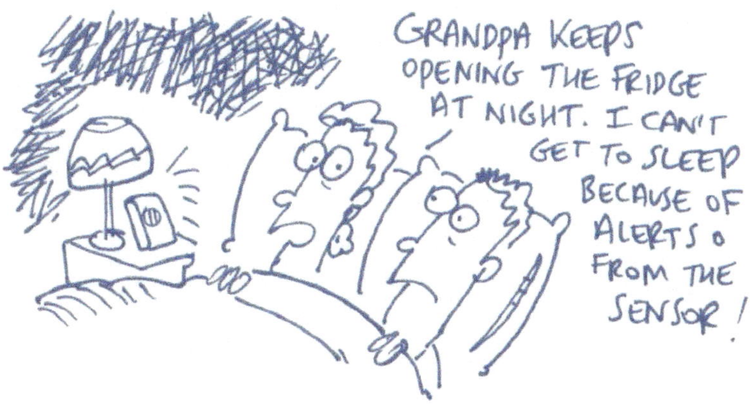
GRANDPA KEEPS OPENING THE FRIDGE AT NIGHT. I CAN'T GET TO SLEEP BECAUSE OF ALERTS FROM THE SENSOR!

Is pain keeping you awake? You could take painkillers for your degenerating joints before you climb into bed, or get the cause seen to by a doctor or physiotherapist.

Keep a sleep diary. Once you know what's causing you to lose sleep, you can tackle the source and hopefully sleep better for it.

Possible treatments to try

Prescribed drugs – best to try to do without them but if you must:

- Drugs like zopiclone are non-benzodiazepine hypnotics. They have a short duration of action – around 4 hours - and should only be used short term, say for four weeks. It's easy to get addicted so only take them on two or three nights a week and for a few consecutive nights every so often. Otherwise you won't sleep with them and you won't be able to sleep without them either. The problem is that you can get rebound insomnia when you stop taking such a drug.
- Benzodiazepine drugs such as temazepam are hypnotic drugs. They can have side effects such as impairing your memory, and dull your sharpness of thinking; and insomnia can restart when you stop taking them. You can get dependent on them pretty quickly; then get into a state where you don't sleep much with them and don't sleep without them. Be careful too - if you're groggy after taking them you could have a fall and hurt yourself in the middle of the night, and even end up with a fracture that could have been avoided.
- A sedating antidepressant like amitryptiline may be worth trying in a small dose at night.

Relaxation

Relaxation seems to help to alleviate sleep problems, maybe relieving stress symptoms that are disturbing someone's sleep. Move through a relaxing sequence before getting into bed. Don't work too late, read quietly, or do some yoga. Have a hot bath and lie and wallow in it. Learn to switch off mentally when you turn off the light. Picture a pleasant scene where you're relaxed.

Relaxation techniques like autogenic training, biofeedback and meditation could help you drop off and sleep better.

Cognitive behavioural therapy (CBT)

CBT does improve sleep quality for some people. The aim is to identify and alter your beliefs and expectations about sleep, and getting to sleep. It can help to reduce your anxiety about not getting enough sleep and the consequences of not sleeping. CBT can be delivered in person, in a group, or digitally via internet or smartphone applications. The interventions are typically delivered in regular weekly sessions over a period of 8-12 weeks. Even as much as a year on after the CBT has finished, your sleep should still be improved.

Digital aids to help you combat sleep problems

Screen time at night is linked to poor sleep as the blue light from digital screens can mess with your sleep cycle, tricking the body into thinking it should be waking up, not going to sleep. Refrain from staring at a screen for a minimum of 30 minutes before going to bed, although the longer the better. If you do use your phone or tablet, then lower the screen brightness. However, technology isn't all bad when it comes to sleep – try some of these if you are struggling to get 40-winks:

Website	Video	App
Thesleepcharity.org.uk	**Sleep pattern discussed**	**MyNoise.net**

Smart speaker

Why not access some breathing exercises just before bed? They can really help to clear your mind and ensure a restful night's sleep.

Video streaming: YouTube has some great white noise videos and scenes. These are very popular and really useful for many people who are struggling to sleep. If you need 10-hours of airplane cabin noise, then YouTube has your back - just remember to turn your screen brightness down to its lowest setting.

Apps

Lots of white noise apps are available with a wide range of soundscapes. The advantages of an app is that there is often a sleep timer option, ensuring that your phone will have stopped making a noise when you're fast asleep.

Online tips on improving your sleep:

https://www.nhs.uk/conditions/insomnia/

https://www.nhs.uk/live-well/sleep-and-tiredness/how-to-get-to-sleep/

Medito meditation app

Look for **Medito** in the Apple App store or Google Play Store

Apple

Playstore

The **Calm** app offers help with meditation and sleep and helps to reduce stress and anxiety, with relaxing music.

Look for 'Calm' on the App Store or Google Play.

Apple

Playstore

Case study

Malcolm had had difficulties sleeping without being disturbed for decades. Then he read the advice that's included in the chapter of this book!! So he took regular exercise – his step count was over 10,000 nearly everyday for six months (that ensured he wasn't taking naps sitting around watching TV too as he was out and about a lot more). He avoided alcohol – well for at least six days of the week, with a treat when he met up with friends on Saturdays.
He switched to having his main meal at lunchtime most days and went for decaffeinated drinks. He turned off his phone at 10pm every night and wore ear plugs so that he couldn't hear his wife snoring next to him (after many years of getting really annoyed by her noise). So guess what? Now he sleeps for seven hours or so every night, with just one break for a toilet stop - not unexpected at his 71 year old age.

Questions and answers

Q1. I was looking forward to a relaxing life once I retired, getting up late, watching daytime TV, having coffee with friends. But now I'm a free agent my days are wrecked as after on/off sleep at night, I catnap through the day. What can I do?

A.Take regular exercise. Getting physically tired should help you to sleep. Try for at least 30 minutes of moderate exercise most or all days of the week. Take a walk every day; or perhaps 20 - 30 minutes of regular swimming or workout in your local or home gym. Avoid alcohol – drinking excessively is out. And no heavy meals in the evening. Avoid caffeine containing drinks – gets your heart racing and keeps you awake. Don't let yourself take catnaps in the day - they'll mess up your sleep pattern.

Q2. I'm scared of getting addicted to sleeping tablets. Are there any complementary treatments that work?

A. There is some evidence that low doses of melatonin can help to improve sleep quality short-term; you might be able to get a prescription for it depending on your age and history of sleep disturbance. Some people do try it for jet lag. Or you could try meditation for a few minutes before bedtime. Relaxation therapy can help alleviate sleep problems too.

Chapter 13. Get tech help if you are feeling low

Top tips

1. You might try psychological and behaviour treatments as well as, or instead of, medication, like:
    a. cognitive behavioural therapy: a 'talking' therapy used for people suffering from depression, anxiety and eating disorders.
    b. problem solving: which is briefer and simpler than cognitive therapy and consists of three stages: (1) identifying your main problems; (2) generating solutions; (3) trying out the solutions – so you don't put up with unnecessary or avoidable pressures.
2. Develop good coping skills. Remember it is not stress itself that is the damaging factor but your inability to cope with it. In a changing world you need to learn new ways of coping. That way lies survival.

Mental ill health is common

At any one time, around one adult in six suffers from one or other form of mental illness – and is probably even more frequent now thanks to the COVID pandemic across the world. Mental ill-health is about as common as asthma. Mental health problems range from common conditions such as work stress, anxiety or depression, to psychotic illnesses such as schizophrenia or bipolar affective disorder (manic depression) that only affect one person in 250. People with mental health problems often suffer from poor physical health too due to them being less likely to strive for a healthy lifestyle and being more likely to have a poor diet, drink excessive alcohol and maybe get adverse effects from their prescribed medication.

Stress

Stress is very difficult to define as it is such a vague word and everyone interprets it differently. One of the secrets of a happy life is to get the balance of stress right. Stress is equivalent to a person's perception of the pressure upon them, or the three way relationship between demands on a person, that person's feelings about those demands and their ability to cope with those demands. So, in other words, a particular event or task can be very stressful for you one day but not on another - all depending on how you are feeling and what other pressures are being exerted on you. And what is stressful for *you* might not be for somebody else, whose perceptions and ways of coping with pressures are different.

In general, work stress occurs in situations where the workload or pressures are high, control over your workload or pressures is limited, and too little is available in the way of support or help for you. It depends on how much stress you are under, for how long it is applied and whether you feel powerless to stand up to the stress or can overcome it. A moderate amount of stress is necessary to perform well and to maintain a zest for life. Zero stress may lead to boredom whereas too much stress over too long a period will render you indecisive, exhausted or burnt out. One of the ways to reduce stress is to timetable enough free time during your day to have space for rest and relaxation to counteract the stresses and strains of your everyday life – which might include pressures at work and your home life bringing up children or supporting a loved one, or maybe financial constraints and worries.

Try and organise your working life (or your everyday life if you are retired) so that you have enough time for non-work related activities. If you do not allow sufficient time for leisure you will not have the opportunity for personal growth and will probably become stale. Every so often, you might set a target to learn or improve at something outside work or take active measures to nurture your relationship with your spouse, family and friends, by sharing a new hobby for example.

The best options are solutions that make regular time and space for yourself for fun, relaxation, hobbies and enjoying simple pleasures throughout your life as a *stress proofing* measure. Don't suddenly try and adopt these methods to beat stress at one particular time in your working life, when you are already under par. One of the best ways of monitoring whether you are managing to protect enough time for yourself is to keep a daily log of activities, for a week or so.

Be honest and indicate how much time you spent in the previous week pursuing an activity that was for *your own* enjoyment.

You might experience personal symptoms of stress including:

- anxiety
- palpitations
- feeling burdened
- insomnia
- panic / hyperventilate
- reduced appetite
- tired / drained
- being jumpy
- difficulty concentrating
- feeling depressed
- nausea / indigestion
- being cynical
- loss of confidence
- lack of self-esteem
- feelings of helplessness.

Or you might behave differently:

- put things off
- be indecisive
- shunt work away
- be less efficient
- be late for work often
- breakdown in relationships
- argumentative
- irritable
- make mistakes
- accident prone
- loss of interest in sex
- overeating.

What about depression?
Depression consists of persistent low mood, loss of interest and enjoyment and reduced energy. It affects the majority of people at some time. Around two-thirds of adults will experience depression or worry of sufficient severity to influence their daily activities at least once in their lives. Episodes of depression are short-lived for most people. Depression can affect other family members too – for example the emotional and cognitive development of socially deprived children who have a depressed mother.

Episodes of 'major' depression are twice as common in women as men. Depression is the most common mental health problem in older people, especially in those living in nursing and residential care. 10-15% of older adults, aged over 65 years old have significant depressive symptoms, although major depression is rare. Women are more likely to be depressed than men. The term 'bipolar' describes depression that occurs in conjunction with manic episodes. Other depression is termed 'unipolar'.

Depression and anxiety often present together. Symptoms include:

- depressed mood
- markedly diminished interest or pleasure in normal activities
- significant weight loss or gain
- insomnia or hypersomnia
- agitated or retarded
- fatigue or loss of energy
- sadness, loss of enjoyment
- feelings of worthlessness or excessive guilt
- negative thoughts or hopelessness, lack of motivation
- guilt, shame, anger
- loss of libido
- social withdrawal
- diminished ability to think or concentrate, poor memory, indecisiveness
- recurrent thoughts of death or suicidal thoughts or actions, self harm

If you answer 'yes' to either or both of the following questions then you may have depression and could consider consulting a doctor:

1. During the past month have you often been bothered by feeling down, depressed or hopeless?
2. During the past month, have you often been bothered by having little interest or pleasure in doing things?

Mild to moderate depression: sufferers have depressive symptoms and some functional impairment – that is, they do not perform as they usually would do. Many recover in the short term, and about half have recurrent symptoms.

Severe depression: sufferers have depressive symptoms plus agitation or psychomotor retardation and somatic symptoms such as muscular aches.

Psychotic depression: sufferers have hallucinations, delusions or both in addition to their depressive symptoms.

How it happens

About half the people who have major depression experience a further depressive episode in the following ten years. Major depression is strongly associated with adverse life and economic circumstances – such as unemployment, divorce or poor housing.

People may have a genetic tendency to depression. Having a family history of depression increases someone's chance of depression in childhood or later life.

People who've experienced poor relationships are more vulnerable to depression – for example, poor parent-child relationships, divorce, physical and sexual abuse etc.

Life events such as bereavement, moving house, changing or losing jobs can trigger depression. Some people who have chronic diseases such as diabetes or stroke or heart disease may become depressed too. People who live in difficult circumstances may have a tendency to depression- for example living in poverty or being unemployed.

With the seasonal affective disorder (SAD) depression is linked to seasonal variations in light, reducing during the autumn and winter months. Typically symptoms begin in the autumn, peak in the winter and get better in the spring.

What you can do yourself to minimise symptoms from depression

- Take regular physical activity: aim for 30 minutes of moderate exercise at least five times a week. It should help to lift your mood
- as well as improving your physique. Exercise outdoors may help lift your mood particularly if you suffer from the SAD syndrome.

- Get a positive outlook. Convince yourself that you can change or improve things through positive thinking. Use positive body language and people will automatically treat you more positively. Try positive visualisation - keep picturing a scene where you do well instead of imagining everything going wrong. Remember past successes. Praise yourself for your successes and achievements; do not focus on your minor imperfections. Challenge any negative thoughts.

- Sometimes people are diagnosed as having depression who are really just 'sad'. Sadness is normal. Sometimes it is 'medicalised' by doctors attaching the depression tag to sad feelings. So if this fits with what's been happening to you, chat your feelings of sadness over with a friend, realise what's causing you to feel sad, and work towards regaining a positive mindset.

- You could give marital therapy a try if your or your partner's depression is associated with your relationship breaking down or you are going through a rocky patch.

- Look after yourself better as far as other health problems go. So if you have diabetes say, and you think that your depression is partly down to that condition, then stick to a sensible diet, take plenty of exercise and follow your doctor's or nurse's advice as far as managing your diabetes goes.

- Develop your social life. If you've cut yourself off from friends, revitalise your relationships with them. Maybe join a club and find people with shared interests.

- Try to restore your sleep if depression has given you sleepless nights.

- Look after yourself with a good diet. Don't drink alcohol excessively or take recreational drugs - that could make you more depressed.

Relax more. To the competitive person, relaxation means doing their usual sport or pastime at a slower speed. Someone else might interpret 'complete' relaxation as being in an entirely passive state away from all pressure and hassles – say on a lounger on a beach. Listening to relaxation tapes can have a soothing and calming influence on one person, and be intensely irritating to another. It all depends on your personal preference and style. Learning to relax whilst visualising events that upset you, can help you to control the feelings provoked in the real situation that usually triggers that stress. Try different forms of relaxation, meditation, yoga or self-hypnosis to find an approach that suits you.

Make sure that there is something positive that can easily be seen from your work desk - or at home maybe over the kitchen sink? A photograph of the family? Perhaps a holiday memento that you associate with happy times could be one of the best methods of transporting you from the stresses of your working life and remind you of the next holiday on your horizon. An award of some sort could be displayed to reinforce the feelings of achievement and being valued.

Good time management will help you to prioritise what is important for you to complete and put your energies into - at work or home.

Playing with a pet can help you to relax and cast cares aside.
The friendship and love from your pet will make you feel generally better and give you a lift, to combat a low mood or stress symptoms.
Research has shown that pets can help to lower your blood pressure and even add years to your life.

A new hobby or special interest should help to distract you from your feelings of stress and their sources, and put things in perspective. Art, drama, music, dance are great ways to relax, build your self confidence, express your emotions that may be bottled up for various reasons.

Positive thinking helps, talking yourself back to a normal state, reassuring yourself that nothing bad happened to you before when you were in a state of panic and you'll feel better again when you calm down. Breathing into a brown paper bag or large envelope if you're in the midst of a panic attack can help sometimes as the exhaled carbon dioxide that you rebreathe instead of fresh air reduces your panicky feelings.

Keep a stress diary: log all the sources of stress in your day for say a week, to cover a typical period, at work, at home, social period and family time. Record your feelings and any symptoms associated with stress and see if you can spot any trends. This will help identify what's causing your stress and then work to minimise the sources of your stress.

Getting motivated

Motivation may be positive or negative. With **positive motivation** you may be stimulated to act differently because of being inspired, or seeing how possible actions might influence your future. You make the most of your urge to achieve things.

With **negative motivation** you may act because you fear failure or punishment or that other adverse events could happen. That threat can be a powerful motivating force for change too.

Positive motivation leads to a deeper understanding and better long-term change than negative motivation. We seek to achieve things, accept challenges, learn different ways of thinking or new skills throughout our lives. Positive factors include wanting to succeed at something, like career goals or better lifestyle habits or other challenge.

Other positive influences include competition, respect for others, not wishing to let the side down and admiring someone. Competition can motivate some people but may de-motivate others.

You must be motivated to change, maybe changing from having risky lifestyle habits to a healthy lifestyle. Start off by contemplating that change and then take action. Set realistic targets for change that are achievable, otherwise you'll be demotivated if you keep failing and find an escape route ("I knew I couldn't do it.").

Possible treatments to try

Prescribed drugs
Antidepressant drugs are effective for moderate to severe depression. Some of these drugs are contraindicated if you have other health problems. Possible side effects such as agitation, nausea/vomiting, weight gain, dizziness, malaise/lassitude, sleep disturbance and headache/migraine vary in the likelihood of happening between different antidepressant drugs. Such side effects often cause some people to stop taking antidepressants, although for most patients, the benefits of treatment far outweigh the risks or adverse effects of their prescribed medication.

Problem solving therapy (for mild to moderate depression)
Most problems have solutions. Work through the following steps. Don't rush; you may need to work through the exercises over a period of time.

1 List all your difficulties and problems.
2 Prioritise the items on your list- which will be the easiest or hardest to solve?
3 Select the problem you will work on first.
4 List all the possible options that you can think of for this problem, from the silliest to the most sensible options.
5 Work out the advantages and disadvantages for each and every option.
6 Pick the option you will work on first. Do not rush into actioning this option. Take time to thing it through. Break the tasks down to achieve the option into small steps that are doable for you.
7 Plan when and where and how you will carry out each of these steps.
8 Now work through the steps with the timetables you have set.
9 How has it been going? If you haven't achieved the successes you needed, go back through the list and work out where it started to go

wrong. This would be a good place to start again, perhaps picking different solutions, or breaking the options down further into more manageable stages. If you have been successful - well done! Now start on the other problems.

Relaxation

Relaxation can help people suffering from depression. Music therapy is a form of relaxation that might help.

Apps in both Apple App Store and Google Playstore

Mood tools
A variety of methods to help improve positive thoughts and overcome depression.

Apple Playstore

Well Mind
Gives advice on stress, anxiety and depression.

Apple Playstore

What's Up?
A Mental Health App uses proven therapy to help with anxiety, depression, anger and stress.

Apple Playstore

My Possible Self helps you take control of feelings, thoughts, habits, to overcome fear, anxiety and stress.

Apple Playstore

Catch it helps you to see how you react to situations, and change your behaviour.

Apple

Playstore

Calm Harm uses various methods to help you overcome the urge to self harm.

Apple

Playstore

Chill Panda helps children use breathing to relax and feel less stressed.

Apple

Playstore

Drinkaware helps you reduce how much alcohol you are drinking.

Apple

Playstore

equoo is an adventure. game to help increase emotional fitness and learn new psychological skills.

Apple

Playstore

Website	Video	App	
Mind.org	**How to manage your mood with food**	**Healthy Minds**	
		Apple	Playstore

Smart Speaker

A brilliant source of information; just a quick question to a smart speaker could help to put your mind at rest about a worrying query you have. Use your smart speaker to help you with breathing techniques, to listen to relaxing music, to gain tips and advice that will help you to relax.

Search term keywords and phrases:

- breathing exercises
- meditation
- relaxing mood
- mental health conditions and associated issues.
- support for money issues, employment, housing and family matters.

Case studies

Ian has finally got over his long-standing depression and anxiety and has been off all treatment for six months. He's in a pressurised job but copes with it well. His secret? He says it's down to his 'sleep hygiene'. He now goes to bed about 10pm every day and gets up at 6am or a bit later at weekends. The regular eight hours sleep has made all the difference. When he wakes up, he's ready for the day and gets up full of gusto. He drinks very little alcohol now too.

Alan was diagnosed as having a bipolar condition in his 20s, thirty years ago. Using the Alexa Echo Show has greatly improved his adherence to his medication through his use of reminders. This has meant that he could move out of supported living to his own accommodation – so he no longer even requires care visits to ensure that he has taken his medication because his adherence is so reliable now.

Questions and answers

Q1. I took an antidepressant last year when my husband died but I started being sick, felt dizzy and got migraines so I stopped taking it. I'm still feeling low, so what else can I do?

A. The symptoms you describe might have been a side effect of your medication, or have been connected with your low mood. You could try a different antidepressant or go for self help from a local support service – look at your local Council's website to see if there is a self-referral service which helps local people with bereavement.

Q2. My daughter's recently had her first baby but instead of being happy to have such a lovely little boy she's sad and weepy. Could this be depression?

A. At least one in ten women experiences depression soon after the birth of a baby. Most recover without any treatment within a few months. But it is definitely worth her seeking help from her GP and health visitor or she may feel down for six months or much longer – and they can help her.

Chapter 14. Evolving your action plan to bring assistive tech into your daily life

The approach to self care that we've emphasised throughout this book is to make the most of the health you've got - minimising your risk factors which might include: being overweight, lack of fitness, drinking too much alcohol, smoking / passive smoking, limited social/family life, low mood, risky hobbies and so preventing deterioration of your health and wellbeing. Maximising your use of digital aids like the apps scattered through this book, and other equipment and devices that are accessible and available can support you in achieving this behaviour change.

So assess how ready you are to change your lifestyle habits and way of life, and ensure that you try to stay fit and mobile, overcome any frailty and poor balance, strengthen your muscles and joints, improve your memory – and plot what help and assistive technology resources you'll need.

You must motivate yourself to optimise your health and wellbeing by harnessing your friends' and family's support, resisting temptations, and finding satisfaction in your everyday life - with consistently healthy habits.

To improve your lifestyle and sustain all these positive benefits long-term means that you must want to change, then progress to preparing to change, and move on to actually making those changes. You may relapse and need encouragement to then repeat the process and sustain the changes you've made to your everyday life and behaviour. So take a look and work through the five stages of the cycle of change below to think through what you need to do to overcome any problems in accomplishing your healthy lifestyle goals and try to stick with your achievements forever.

So off you go......begin to build your action plan to identify your resource needs to lead a happy, safe and independent life; describing where you are now, what your goals are, how you are going to reach those goals and sustain your improved life.

Your five stages of change

Pre-contemplation: you've no intention to change your behaviour in the foreseeable future.

So even if you are overweight, or sitting down for most of the day, or just about managing in your everyday life.....you're oblivious to any risks or don't really care........or don't see the benefits.........

So now describe your current thinking about the life you're living, if you're oblivious or are not particularly bothered about the state of your daily life or independence or health and wellbeing:

Contemplation: you are aware of the problems that exist and are seriously thinking about overcoming them but have not yet made a commitment to take action.

So you're thinking of what changes you might take to your lifestyle and daily living....maybe reading or hearing good stories of how other people have made successful changes to their lives that you could mirror?

So now describe your current thinking about any problems that you are aware of in your daily life or independence or health and wellbeing, what changes you would like to make, and how and when that might be:

Preparation: you are intending to take action in the next few days or months and (may) have unsuccessfully taken action in the past year.

So get ready.....steady......go. You've read this book avidly, absorbing all the useful information in each chapter that relates to you - such as the assistive tech that might help you, the answers to the questions that you had too and the successful case studies at the end of each chapter.
So now think out what changes you'll make to your everyday living and home or work environment, and what products and assistive aids you'll need to buy, and what skills you'll need to be more confident to use technology, digital aids like apps and personal assistants, and assistive equipment and devices for your daily life.

So now describe what actions you plan to take and changes you hope to make in relation to the state of your daily life or independence or health and wellbeing – what/when/how, and describe what you will need to buy or access or learn too:

Action: you are now modifying your behaviour, experiences, or environment (including products such as equipment and devices you now have access to) in order to overcome your weaknesses, and build these changes into your daily life with obvious benefits to your health and wellbeing, independence and safety.

So now describe the actions you have taken to improve the life you're living, and boost your health and wellbeing (be as specific as you can, describing how confident you now are in using technology, digital aids like apps and personal assistants, and assistive equipment and devices in your daily life):

Maintenance: you are working hard so as not to relapse; you're consolidating the gains you've attained.

So now describe the actions you have taken to sustain your improved lifestyle and habits that boost your health and wellbeing (be as specific as you can, describing your use of technology, digital aids like apps and personal assistants, and assistive equipment and devices in your daily life). What further developments are you adopting or planning to maintain the positive changes to your lifestyle and habits – what/why/when/how?

Keep it up!

Printed in Great Britain
by Amazon

65802412R00098